12/16

Drug Dealer, M

DRUG DEALER, MD

How Doctors Were Duped,
Patients Got Hooked,
and Why It's So Hard to Stop

ANNA LEMBKE, MD

JOHNS HOPKINS UNIVERSITY PRESS | *Baltimore*

© 2016 Johns Hopkins University Press
All rights reserved. Published 2016
Printed in the United States of America on acid-free paper
9 8 7 6 5 4 3 2 1

Johns Hopkins University Press
2715 North Charles Street
Baltimore, Maryland 21218-4363
www.press.jhu.edu

Library of Congress Cataloging-in-Publication Data

Names: Lembke, Anna, 1967–
Title: Drug dealer, MD : how doctors were duped, patients got hooked, and why it's so
    hard to stop / Anna Lembke, MD.
Description: Baltimore : Johns Hopkins University Press, 2016. | Includes
    bibliographical references and index.
Identifiers: LCCN 2016010031 | ISBN 9781421421407 (pbk. : alk. paper) | ISBN
    1421421402 (pbk. : alk. paper) | ISBN 9781421421414 (electronic) | ISBN
    1421421410 (electronic)
Subjects: LCSH: Analgesics. | Medication abuse. | Physician and patient. | Drugs—
    Prescribing. | Drug addiction.
Classification: LCC RM319 .L46 2016 | DDC 615.7/83—dc23
    LC record available at http://lccn.loc.gov/2016010031

A catalog record for this book is available from the British Library.

*Special discounts are available for bulk purchases of this book. For more information, please
contact Special Sales at 410-516-6936 or specialsales@press.jhu.edu.*

Johns Hopkins University Press uses environmentally friendly book materials,
including recycled text paper that is composed of at least 30 percent post-consumer
waste, whenever possible.

To every patient who has been addicted to prescription drugs, to their loved ones, and to all the doctors who went into medicine to do good but feel trapped by a system gone awry

Contents

Acknowledgments

This book would not have been possible without my patients' willingness to share their stories. I thank them for their generosity and courage. I also thank the many health care professionals who agreed to be interviewed; their experiences and perspectives lend richness and texture to my own.

I've had many wonderful teachers over the years. I am especially grateful to Keith Humphreys and John Ruark, who have guided me, challenged me, and always rooted for me.

Several people have read all or parts of the manuscript along the way. My thanks to my editors Robin W. Coleman and Barbara Lamb and to several anonymous reviewers for Johns Hopkins University Press. Special thanks to my mother-in-law, Jean Chu, one of my earliest readers, a fantastic editor, and a dear friend.

My deepest gratitude to my husband and children, for allowing me time and relative quiet to work on "the book."

Note on Terminology

The terminology to refer to people who use drugs and become addicted to drugs is in flux. There is increased awareness, especially among treatment providers, that the language currently used to describe addiction stigmatizes the people involved. Examples include calling someone who is in recovery "clean," as if they were "dirty" before; referring to addictive drug use as "drug abuse," which conjures images of other forms of abuse, such as child abuse; or referring to the addicted individual as a "drunk" or a "junkie."

Throughout this book, I have attempted to avoid stigmatizing language in favor of more neutral terms, such as "use," "misuse," "overuse" "addictive use," and "addiction." Nonetheless, terms like "addict," "drunk," and "junkie" do appear in this book, when patients themselves use these words to describe their behavior and experiences. Indeed, in the twelve-step self-help community (Alcoholics Anonymous, Narcotics Anonymous, etc.), members often refer to themselves as "alcoholic drug addicts." My use of these terms is hence not meant to be pejorative, but to capture the language and experience of drug-addicted individuals.

Drug Dealer, MD

Prologue

After I finished medical school in 1995, followed by a residency in psychiatry and a fellowship in mood disorders (an apprenticeship period that follows medical school), I was finally ready, after nearly ten years of medical training, to treat patients on my own. As I was establishing my clinic at the academic medical center that hired me, I informed the intake coordinators (who check insurance, do a brief psychiatric assessment by phone, and triage patients to the appropriate clinic) that I wouldn't see anyone addicted to drugs or alcohol.

My reluctance in those days to treat patients with substance* use issues was consistent with my training. I received no education in medical school on the treatment of addiction, and limited education on addiction even during my residency in psychiatry. I was schooled to believe that addiction is not a medical disorder and, therefore, not treatable in the traditional sense. My teachers never mentioned existing pharmacotherapy and behavioral interventions for substance use

* "Substance" is the generally accepted medical term for any addictive chemical. "Substance use disorder" is the term for addiction found in the American Psychiatric Association's *Diagnostic and Statistical Manual of Mental Disorders*.

disorders. I acquired no skills on how to talk with patients about the often thorny issue of harmful substance use. Alcoholics Anonymous was mentioned, but outside of being encouraged to observe an AA meeting as a guest, no education was provided on how AA might be helpful to patients.

I soon discovered that, despite my effort to avoid treating patients with substance use problems, many of my patients were either misusing or addicted to a variety of substances. According to national surveys, 75 percent or more of patients with mental illness struggle with drug and/or alcohol problems.[1] I became aware of my patients' substance use not through any clinical prowess or discernment of my own. To the contrary, in the 1990s I seldom if ever asked my patients about drug or alcohol use. Instead, I typically came into this knowledge after a desperate call from the patient's family member, along the lines of: "Holly has been in a rollover car accident. Didn't you know that she shoots up heroin every day?!" No, I was forced to admit, despite being her psychiatrist, I really hadn't known—mostly because I hadn't thought to ask.

By the late 1990s, I realized I had one of two choices: I could continue to ignore my patients' substance use problems or I could figure out how to target and treat addiction. Out of necessity I chose the latter. It became increasingly clear to me that my patients were not going to get better otherwise. Then began a period of reeducation for me. For the next ten years, with the guidance of wonderful colleagues already versed in addiction treatment, and the insight, and sometimes lack of insight, of my patients—who proved to be the best teachers of all—I learned what addiction is, how to detect it, and how to intervene to help patients struggling with it. By default, I became the go-to person in my department for patients with substance use disorders. In addition to alcohol, tobacco, and marijuana, I saw increasing numbers of patients addicted to prescription drugs.

The majority of my patients who were misusing prescription drugs were *not* getting their drugs from a drug dealer; they were getting them from a doctor. Sometimes I was the unwitting prescriber. The extent of the problem was brought home to me in 2011, when I was asked to see a patient admitted to the hospital for severe low back pain. My colleagues consulted me to determine whether the patient was addicted to opioids.*

According to this patient's medical records, her history was marked by the classic downward spiral of a drug-ravaged life, including loss of jobs, friends, family, and a recent near-death opioid overdose. In the months prior to admission, she had obtained and presumably taken more than 1,200 different opioid pills obtained from sixteen different doctors.

I went to see the patient. I heard her before I met her, her demands for more painkillers ricocheting off the walls of the hospital hallway. Her nurses hovered outside her door, afraid to enter, a look of panic in their eyes. When I walked in, the patient saw my white coat and seemed relieved. She launched into her story of unbearable pain. She also freely admitted being addicted to opioids in any form, from prescription painkillers to intravenous heroin. But to her this presented no obstacle to obtaining more pain medication: "I know I'm addicted, Doc, but if you don't give me the pills I want, I'll sue you for leaving me in pain."

I realized then that we—I and my fellow health care providers—had become trapped in a system gone mad. We were unable to deny this obviously addicted patient more opioid painkillers, even when we were well aware of the harm these medications were causing her. I recom-

---

* Opioids (o-pee-oyds) are powerful painkillers (pain relievers) used for centuries to relieve pain. Opioids work by binding opioid receptors in the brain and blocking pain signals. We have opioid receptors in our brains because we make our own opioids, called endorphins, to block pain. Endorphins work only for minutes at a time, whereas the newly synthesized pain relievers like OxyContin, work for many hours, and bind the opioid receptor more strongly. Originally derived from the poppy plant as opium, many opioids today are synthesized, or partially synthesized, in the laboratory. By changing the chemical composition of naturally occurring opioids, scientists work to create new and better opioids to treat pain. Their efforts have also been driven by the goal of creating an opioid that targets pain without creating addiction. These efforts have met with mixed results.

mended to my colleagues that they slowly discontinue her opioid pain-killers and refer her to addiction treatment. None of my recommendations were followed, and high-dose opioid painkillers were continued for the length of her hospital stay. When she presented to the hospital again a month later, with the same complaint of pain, she received the same treatment. All of us were caught on a merry-go-round that we felt helpless to stop.

A Prescription Drug Epidemic

This patient's care was not an aberration. Her case was emblematic of a new normal. On November 1, 2011, the Centers for Disease Control and Prevention (CDC), the agency of the government responsible for protecting Americans from major health threats, declared a "prescription drug epidemic"; and the CDC was unequivocal about what had caused this epidemic: "prescription opioid painkillers and psychotherapeutic drugs being prescribed more widely by physicians."[2] In the United States, approximately 4,000 deaths involving opioid painkillers were documented in 1999,[3] increasing to 16,235 in 2013,[4] quadrupling in little more than a decade. The combination of opioid painkillers and sedative benzodiazepines (for example, Valium) has contributed to a large number of the overdose deaths.[5,6]

Pharmacy retail sales of opioid painkillers, obtained through doctors' prescriptions, quadrupled between 1999 and 2010,[7] coinciding with a quadrupling in prescription-opioid-related deaths. Prescribers wrote enough opioid painkiller prescriptions in 2012 to medicate every American adult around the clock for a month. Equally alarming has been the increased prescribing of stimulants (for example, Adderall) and sedatives (for example, Xanax) over the last three decades.

By 2010, for the first time in history, unintentional drug poisonings represented the leading cause of injury death in the United States, exceeding deaths due to motor vehicle accidents.[7] The total toll of prescription opioid overdoses between 1999 and 2013 exceeded 175,000 lives. This scourge did not discriminate, crossing every geographic and racial boundary, with the largest increases among middle-class whites living in nonurban areas.[8]

Scheduled (Controlled) Prescription Drugs

The drugs posing the greatest risk for misuse, overuse, and addiction are the "scheduled" (controlled) drugs.

The Food and Drug Administration (FDA), working under the Controlled Substance Act (CSA), has organized a subset of prescription drugs into a category called "scheduled drugs." Scheduled drugs are drugs that have the potential for addiction and/or physiologic dependence. The FDA has delineated a grading system from one to five within the scheduled drugs, with schedule I drugs being the most addictive and schedule V drugs the least addictive. All drugs in schedules II through V are thought to have medical benefit in some situations and can be prescribed by a doctor with a special license. Schedule I drugs, according to federal classification, have no medical benefit and thus cannot be prescribed by a doctor under any circumstances.

Examples of schedule I drugs include heroin, lysergic acid diethylamide (LSD), 3,4-methylenedioxymethamphetamine ("Ecstasy"), and —brace yourself—marijuana. Despite federal classification of marijuana as a schedule I drug, it is widely available in more than twenty states through medical marijuana dispensaries, putting state and federal regulations in direct opposition.

Schedule II drugs include most of the opioid painkillers. Doctors can typically give no more than a month's worth of schedule II medication at a time, with no refills allowed. Examples include morphine, opium, codeine, hydrocodone (brand name Vicodin), hydromorphone (Dilaudid), methadone (Dolophine), meperidine (Demerol), oxycodone (OxyContin, Percocet), and fentanyl (Sublimaze, Duragesic). Vicodin and similar products were reclassified from schedule III to schedule II with the Safe Prescribing Act of 2013, in recognition of the widespread misuse of Vicodin products in the 1990s and 2000s.

Stimulants, which are also considered to be highly addictive, are in schedule II. They are most often used in the treatment of attention deficit hyperactivity disorder (ADHD) and include amphetamines (Dexedrine, Adderall) and methylphenidate (Ritalin).

Schedule III includes buprenorphine (Suboxone), ketamine, and anabolic steroids such as Depo-Testosterone. Doctors can provide limited refills of these medications with one prescription, unlike schedule II drugs.

Schedule IV drugs include the important subgroup of the sedative hypnotics, so-named because of their use in the treatment of anxiety and insomnia. Benzodiazepines are a class of drug within the sedative-hypnotics, including but not limited to alprazolam (Xanax), clonazepam (Klonopin), diazepam (Valium), lorazepam (Ativan), midazolam (Versed), and temazepam (Restoril). Examples of other schedule IV drugs are carisoprodol (Soma) and zolpidem (Ambien).

Schedule V drugs consist primarily of preparations containing limited quantities of opioids. Examples of schedule V drugs include cough preparations containing not more than 200 mg of codeine per 100 ml (Robitussin AC, Phenergan with Codeine).

The majority of prescription drugs remain unscheduled because they are deemed nonaddictive. However, an unscheduled drug can become scheduled if, over time, its addictive potential comes to light. Such was the case with tramadol, a centrally acting painkiller first approved as an unscheduled drug for use in the United States in 1995 under the name Ultram. The Drug Abuse Warning Network (DAWN), a federally operated national surveillance system that monitors trends in drug-related emergency department visits, reported a 165 percent increase—more than 12,000 cases—in drug-related emergency department visits mentioning tramadol from 1995 to 2002.[9] In 2014, the Drug

Enforcement Agency (DEA) rescheduled tramadol to a schedule IV drug,[10] thereby communicating its addictive potential to doctors and consumers. Tramadol when first ingested has limited opioid painkiller properties, but it is quickly metabolized by the body into a more potent, and hence addictive, opioid painkiller.

A Tangled Web

This book is my attempt to understand how well-meaning doctors across America—most of whom became doctors in the first place to save lives and alleviate suffering—ended up prescribing pills that are killing their patients, and how their patients, seeking treatment for illness and injury, ended up addicted to the very pills meant to save them. More importantly, why do we keep prescribing and consuming these dangerous drugs, even though we know better?

In writing this book I have drawn upon my twenty years of clinical experience seeing patients, as a psychiatrist and an addiction medicine specialist. I have also conducted interviews nationwide with doctors, nurses, pharmacists, social workers, hospital administrators, insurance company executives, journalists, economists, and advocates, as well as patients and their families.

The chapters that follow are framed around the story of my patient Jim. Jim's story encapsulates the enormity and complexity of the prescription drug problem. It spans the period of time before and after a major crackdown on prescribing opioid painkillers, reflecting how some of our attempts to address this epidemic have helped, whereas others have led to new problems. The stories of other patients—Justin, Karen, Sally, Macy, and Diana—are interspersed throughout, in varying degrees of depth and detail, in what I intend as useful digressions to illustrate or elaborate on certain aspects of the prescription drug epidemic. The stories are true; only the names have been changed. My patients have given me permission to share their stories with you.

What I have discovered in the course of my work is that doctors and their patients are caught in a web not entirely of their own making, compelled by forces beyond their control to overprescribe and overconsume prescription drugs. Only by teasing apart the strands of this web can we untangle it and find a way out.

1

What Is Addiction, Who's at Risk, and How Do People Recover?

Born in sun-speckled California in 1952, Jim learned how to drink from his father, a "three-martini-lunch" man who preferred his liquor served up dry from a tall bottle of Old Grand-Dad bourbon whiskey. Jim remembers that bottle, taller than your average whiskey bottle, with a picture of a dapper older fly fisherman on the label, a rod in his lap, a raised glass of whiskey in his hand, and just a hint of mischief in his smiling eyes.

Jim's parents owned a San Francisco Yellow Cab company. His mother worked the cage, assigning rides, tracking fares, keeping the books. His dad's job?—going to lunch. Jim's dad dressed up every morning in a suit and tie and met the "boys" at the local watering hole. Jim believes this division of labor suited his parents. His dad was someone who "liked being taken care of," and he had a special knack for finding people who enjoyed doing just that.

When Jim was 14, his dad started taking him to the occasional lunch, where he got to sit on a high stool and listen to the older men talk. He got his own drink, too. He couldn't "put away" three martinis yet, but he might get through one in an afternoon. Years before the word "alcoholic" became part of Jim's vocabulary, and decades before Jim would look back and realize his father had been one, his dad was his hero.

After high school, Jim attended the Lincoln School of Technology, where he learned automotive repair. When he graduated, his dad helped him acquire an auto shop. It was the 1970s, and awareness of greenhouse gases was taking off in California. Jim figured that smog testing was going to be a huge unmet need in the Bay Area, so he decided to sit for his smog-testing license exam. Jim studied hard for the smog-control certification test, and when he found out he had passed, his father was the first person he told.

"This," his father declared, "is cause for celebration."

Jim's dad was good friends with the local chief of police, a prominent man in the community who, more importantly, owned an RV. To honor Jim's accomplishment, Jim, his dad, the chief, and another friend, Kenny, drove from the Bay Area to the Monterey Peninsula for a weekend of golf. To be specific, the chief drove the RV while the other men sat in the back and drank. They drank from the first turn of the wheel out of the driveway, through every green on the golf course, and all the way home again.

One moment in particular about that trip stands out in Jim's memory. The chief was driving. Jim, his dad, and Kenny were sitting in the back, pleasantly drunk. Jim thought about his exam score and his new automotive repair shop. He looked around at the RV, with its shag carpet, foldaway couch and table, and swivel chairs, complete with plaid upholstery and a cup holder for his Schlitz—not to mention the bathroom and the kitchen right there in the car—and he experienced a deep sense of well-being and hopefulness about the future. "My life is perfect," he thought, "real first class."

Jim spent the next twenty years trying to recapture that moment.

In no time Jim's business was booming, with back-to-back appointments for smog testing all day long. He was making money and growing the business. He started drinking every day. Contrary to the myth that heavy substance use is always a way of coping with life's challenges, that is, some form of self-medication,[11] Jim's alcohol use escalated when his life was going well. At first he was just drinking in the evenings, but before long he started going to the bar around the corner at lunchtime, spending most of the afternoon there and skipping appointments at the shop.

There were still mostly good times in those early days, like the time a Rolls Royce broke down in front of his shop and the owner left it with Jim for a day to be repaired. Jim fixed it, then called up his cousin, a dead ringer for Hank Aaron, and told him to get over to the shop as fast as he could. He called the guys at the bar to let them know Hank Aaron was in his shop and coming over to sign autographs. When Jim's buddies saw "Hank" step out of that Rolls, they broke out in whoops and hollers. It wasn't till an hour into drinking that they guessed the truth, but by then it didn't much matter that they'd been had.

As time went on, Jim's drinking began to adversely impact his physical health and his business. He was waking up in the morning with the shakes, already craving the time when he could take his first drink of the day. The shop was becoming disorganized and Jim more unreliable. After less than a decade, Jim was forced to sell the business for nothing more than parts. As he put it, "I drank the business away." He wasn't yet 30 years old.

After losing his business, Jim took a job at his parents' Yellow Cab company, fixing the cabs that came in for repair. His drinking was unchanged, but the pressures of running a business were gone. As the owner's son, he got special treatment. No one commented if he showed up late or left early. By his own admission, "A lot of people covered for me and I got away with doing a lot less work." Instead of repairing cars, he was spending most of his time at the Green Hills Country Club in Millbrae, where his father, a member, helped get him a membership of his own. As Jim describes the club, "It was a bar with a golf course attached."

Jim made a group of friends at the golf club, all of whom were heavy drinkers like himself. They'd play a round of golf together, and winners would buy drinks. Then losers would buy drinks. Then, "chipmunks would buy drinks." At that time, neither Jim nor his many drinking buddies at the golf club would have identified themselves as having a drinking problem.

As Jim moved into his early forties, he no longer felt safe to drive himself home from the club. He'd been driving drunk for years but had never felt unsafe before. Now even he recognized that he was often too drunk to drive. He'd go around the golf club looking to bum a ride, but pretty soon his friends were making excuses not to drive him home.

Jim managed to get home somehow, and once there, he'd collapse into bed in an alcohol-fueled haze. When he woke in the morning, he'd struggle to remember where his car was. Had he driven himself home, or had someone given him a ride? When he couldn't find his car parked on the street outside his house, he'd call up one of the drivers from the cab company to give him a ride to the club. He frequently found himself standing alone at ten in the morning in a nearly empty parking lot next to his abandoned car.

Jim was running out of friends. He was running out of money. Most importantly, alcohol just wasn't working for him the way it used to. He kept trying to recapture that peak experience when he was 22, traveling in the RV to play golf at the coast. But no matter what he drank, how much he drank, or who he drank with, he just couldn't re-create it. After nearly twenty-five years of regular heavy use, drinking alcohol went from being a purely pleasurable experience for him to being something he did in solitary misery.

Around the time Jim turned 47 years old, his closest buddy at the country club died of an alcohol-cocaine overdose. Jim, who had already begun to think seriously about quitting drinking, had new motivation. He didn't want to die. But how to stop? He couldn't imagine it.

Across the street lived a man Jim affectionately called "Larry the Limey." Larry was a British World War II Air Force veteran and a self-declared "reformed drunk," actively involved in Alcoholics Anonymous, or AA. One day Larry approached Jim and simply said, "Jim, there's a better way." He invited Jim to attend his all-male Wednesday night AA meeting, and Jim went.

Jim instantly hated AA. "What am I doing here in this lonely dungeon of drunks, when someone like me should be sitting on a bar stool at the Green Hills Country Club?" But despite Jim's aversion to affiliating with "drunks," and his sense that he wasn't one of them, he decided, as a kind of experiment, that he would go, just to see what it was like. Sometimes he showed up intoxicated, which was okay with the other men and consistent with AA membership requirements, which asks only that potential members come to meetings with the "desire to stop drinking." To his surprise, Jim discovered that more Wednesdays than not, when he went to an AA meeting, he didn't drink. In between he was still spending most of his time intoxicated. Jim became a fixture at Larry the Limey's all-male Wednesday night meetings, and when he turned 50, Jim decided to walk away from booze for good. "It was the hardest thing I ever had to do, and AA made it possible."

The first year after Jim stopped drinking, he was surprised at how much better he felt. He starting exercising, and although he continued to go to the country club on an almost daily basis, he was spending his time improving his golf game instead of sitting in the bar. He went back to playing the drums, a hobby from his teenage years. He bought a new drum set and even joined a band. He also felt a terrific sense of freedom in those early years of sobriety: he could finally go out to places where they didn't serve alcohol and spend time with people who didn't drink and still have an okay time.

His parents sold the Yellow Cab company, but he was kept on as general manager because his work performance, once he had stopped drinking, was exemplary. He spent more time with his wife and kids, whom he'd largely neglected until then, even as he tolerated his regret about not having been there for them earlier. It was a new millennium, and life was good, and it would continue to be good for a decade. That is, until prescription painkillers found Jim.

What Is Addiction?

In contemporary Western medicine, doctors rely on the *Diagnostic and Statistical Manual of Mental Disorders* (*DSM*), a compendium of many different types of mental illness, to diagnose addiction (substance use disorders*).[12] The *DSM* diagnostic criteria for addiction can be remembered simply as the three "C's": control, compulsion, and consequences. Control refers to out-of-control use, especially using more of a substance than intended. Compulsion refers to spending a great deal of time, energy, and thought (mental real estate) obtaining, using, and recovering from the use of substances. Consequences refers to the social, legal, economic, interpersonal, and moral or spiritual repercussions of continuing to use. According to these diagnostic criteria, Jim was certainly addicted to alcohol, with out-of-control use (drinking until he couldn't drive himself home), compulsive use (progressing to daily drinking), and consequential use (losing his smog testing business).

Jim also manifested the physiologic phenomena associated with, but not necessary for, a diagnosis of addiction: dependence and withdrawal. Physiologic dependence is the process whereby the body comes to rely on the drug to maintain biochemical equilibrium. When the drug is not available at expected doses or time intervals, the body becomes biochemically dysregulated, which manifests as the signs and symptoms of withdrawal. Withdrawal is the physiologic manifestations of not having the substance, the symptoms of which vary from substance to substance. As a general albeit oversimplified principle, the charac-

---

* The language of addiction is in flux, and some people argue that the term "addiction" should be used only to describe the more severe forms of substance use disorder. Furthermore, not all addictive disorders involve substances, for example, sex, gambling, and Internet addictions. Nonetheless, for simplicity's sake, I use "addiction" here interchangeably with "substance use disorders."

teristics of withdrawal from a given substance will be the opposite of intoxication for that substance. For example, intoxication with alcohol includes euphoria, relaxation, lowered heart rate, lowered blood pressure (mild), and sedation (sleep). Withdrawal from alcohol includes dysphoria (unhappiness), agitation, restlessness or tremor, increased heart rate, elevated blood pressure, and insomnia. Even in the absence of physiologic withdrawal, cessation of all addictive substances after sustained habitual use is characterized by insomnia, dysphoria, irritability, or anxiety. In the case of withdrawal from some substances, for example alcohol, seizure and even death are a possibility.[13]

According to neuroscientists, addiction is a disorder of the brain's reward circuitry. Survival of the species depends on maximizing pleasure (finding food when hungry, for example) and minimizing pain (avoiding noxious stimuli). Seeking out pleasure and avoiding pain is adaptive and healthy. The intense pleasure experienced with addictive drugs,[14] and importantly the memory of those pleasurable experiences[15] and the desire to re-create them, is what prompts reuse. Jim's magical RV ride after passing his exam is a prime example of this. Indeed, many people who later go on to develop a substance use disorder describe a vivid positive experience with their early exposure to drugs or alcohol.

If only the brain's reward circuitry would continue to respond the way it does the first time. Unfortunately, with sustained heavy use, the brain undergoes biochemical changes that keep the substance from having its desired effect, and the individual needs more and more to get the same response (tolerance).[16, 17] The individual who is vulnerable to addiction will commit all available resources to obtaining more of the substance, overcoming tolerance, and re-creating its original effect, even forgoing natural rewards like food, finding a mate, or raising children. Over time the substance itself is mistaken as necessary for survival.[14] (For more on the neuroadaptation of addiction, see chapter 5.)

Context and culture also play a role in diagnosing drug and alcohol use disorders.[18] Cross-cultural studies readily demonstrate many "wet" cultures across the world whose members drink as much or more than

Jim and his golf buddies were drinking but which do not consider such behavior pathological.[19] Some ethnographers claim that addictive alcohol consumption does not occur to a significant extent in small-scale preindustrial societies.[20]

Who's at Risk?

A perennial question about addiction is why some people exposed to drugs and alcohol can use them in moderation without ill effects, whereas others go on to become addicted, with all the tragic and often life-threatening consequences that entails. Although no one knows for sure what causes addiction, decades of accumulated evidence point to certain risk factors, which can broadly be divided into three categories: nature, nurture, and neighborhood.

Nature. There is good evidence that vulnerability to addiction is heritable, passed down within a person's genetic code from one generation to the next. The data show that having a biological relative (parent or grandparent) with addiction increases the risk of becoming addicted, and that genetics accounts for between 50 and 70 percent of that risk,[21] a high percentage compared to the currently known genetic contribution in other mental disorders such as depression (30 percent).[22] Genetic risk for addiction appears to be independent of upbringing, as shown by adoption studies of children raised outside the drug-using home.

The mechanism by which vulnerability to addiction is passed down in the genetic code is not known and is likely to involve complex genetics, dependent on many genes coding for different traits. Emotion dysregulation (experiencing emotions with more intensity and for longer than average duration) and impulsivity (the tendency to act on thoughts or emotions without weighing the consequences) have both been shown to be highly heritable traits,[23] and are associated with the later development of addiction.[23-26] Iacono and others have described addiction as an interaction between two neural systems, one that communicates the rewarding properties of an object and another that allows for reflective rather than impulsive behavior.[23]

One way to think about this is to imagine the brain as a car, with a gas pedal and a brake. The limbic system, the emotion processing part of the brain, is the gas pedal, propelling the individual to action and motion. The frontal lobe, the future-planning part of the brain, is the car's brakes, telling the individual when to slow down, stop, and reevaluate. Addiction appears to arise from a fundamental problem in the brain's ability to control its gas pedal and/or its brakes, usually along the lines of too much gas and faulty brakes.

Nurture. We know that children raised in families where using addictive substances is modeled and even encouraged, are at increased risk of developing a substance use disorder,[27] as in Jim's family. Substance use is more likely to occur in adolescents who affiliate with so-called deviant peers.[28] Early childhood trauma increases the risk of addiction. High conflict between parent and child, lack of parental involvement in the child's life, and lack of parental monitoring,[29, 30] also appear to be developmental risk factors.[31, 32] By contrast, Jim's parents were supportive, loving, and actively engaged in his life. Paradoxically, in his case, his close relationship with his father, a heavy drinker, may have complicated Jim's relationship with alcohol, contributing to his own later struggles with addiction.

Neighborhood. The risk of substance use, and hence the development of a substance use disorder, is strongly related to the sheer availability of addictive substances. If an individual lives in a neighborhood where drugs are sold on the street corner, that individual is more likely to experiment with, and get addicted to, those drugs. The classic example of this is American soldiers in Vietnam, many of whom used heroin regularly while in Vietnam, but stopped or greatly curtailed their use after returning to the United States.[33]

This risk factor has particular relevance for today's prescription drug epidemic. The increased availability in the 1990s and 2000s to addictive drugs through a doctor's prescription, suddenly increased the risk of addiction to a growing population of patients being prescribed these drugs, not to mention the larger population with access to these drugs through friends and family members.

According to the July 2014 *Morbidity and Mortality Weekly Report*, US prescribers wrote 82.5 opioid painkiller prescriptions and 37.6 benzodiazepine prescriptions per 100 persons in 2012.[34] Data compiled by the Substance Abuse and Mental Health Services Administration show that the majority of misused prescription drugs is obtained directly or indirectly from a doctor's prescription; only 4 percent of persons misusing or addicted to prescription drugs reports getting them from a drug dealer or a stranger.[35] A study in *The Journal of Pain* (2012) showed that the number one predictor of rates of opioid prescribing in a given geographic region in the United States is the number of available physicians, unrelated to the prevalence of injuries, surgeries, or other conditions requiring treatment for pain.[36]

How Do People Recover from Addiction?

How do people stop using substances once they have become addicted to them? The neuroscientist Roy Wise, who studies addiction in animals, says that the only way an addicted animal will stop using drugs is if the drug is no longer available, the animal is too physically exhausted to administer the drug, or the animal dies.[17] Humans are clearly different from animals, and complex psychological, social, and spiritual factors play a role in the decision to initiate as well as to stop using substances. Jim was indeed getting exhausted, but he wasn't near death, and alcohol was still freely available. Jim believes joining AA made the difference in his case.

Three decades of accumulated scientific evidence demonstrate that AA works[37]—not for everybody, and not all of the time, but those who participate in AA get as much benefit or more as those who receive professionally administered treatments like cognitive behavioral therapy and motivational enhancement therapy, and at a much lower cost, because AA is free.[38] One of the ways AA works is by changing social networks. AA changes behavior through facilitating social contacts with supportive, nondrinking peers, that is, reducing pro-drinking influences and providing abstinent role models.[39] For a gregarious man like Jim, this makes sense. When Jim gave up drinking, he was not just giving up alcohol. He was also giving up his earliest and most fundamental conceptualization of how men socialize with other men. AA provided a solution to this problem: an alternative social network in which drinking didn't occur. It was probably not insignificant that Jim's first introduction to AA was an all-male group.

But AA and other self-help groups for addiction don't work for everyone, and they are not the only way. Some patients do better with individual therapy. Some do better with medication. Most end up using some combination thereof. And some patients recover on their own, with no professional or self-help group intervention at all.[40] What is increasingly clear is that addiction for many is a life-long struggle, requiring life-long treatment or monitoring.

2

Prescription Drugs as the New Gateway to Addiction

In 2012, when Jim turned 60, he developed an infection in his lower back. He went to the Emergency Department at a Bay Area hospital, where he was admitted and given intravenous antibiotics to fight the infection. He also received intravenous morphine, an opioid, to fight the pain.

Jim experienced immediate pain relief from the intravenous morphine, and something else—that sense of well-being that he remembered so well from his early days of alcohol, an energized but peaceful clear-headedness, without worry or doubt. He was instantly under its power.

The rapidity with which Jim became addicted to morphine—possibly after a single dose—speaks to the phenomena of reinstatement and cross-addiction. Neuroscientists speculate that brain changes that occur after continuous heavy use of addictive substances can cause damage that does not resolve even after years of abstinence. One of the ways these irreversible changes can manifest is that the brain is primed to relapse to addictive physiology even after a single exposure to the addictive substance.[41] This is called "reinstatement" by neurobiologists, and "relapse" by those who are addicted.

Reinstatement is not triggered solely by the substance that the individual was previously addicted to. Reinstatement can occur with any addictive substance because all addictive drugs work on the same brain reward pathway.[42] For example, animals repeatedly exposed to the addictive component of marijuana (tetrahydrocannabinol, or THC) and then not given THC for a period of time become addicted to morphine more quickly than animals not previously exposed to THC.[43] This phenomenon is called cross-sensitization, or cross-addiction. The intense high and craving that Jim experienced after a single dose of morphine was likely the result, at least in part, of reinstatement and cross-addiction.

Although a history of addiction increases the risk of becoming addicted to opioid painkillers prescribed by a doctor,[44] many people with no addiction history can become addicted to opioid painkillers in the course of routine medical treatment.[45] Furthermore, they can become addicted quickly, in a matter of days to weeks, just as Jim did. This is contrary to what doctors were told in the 1980s, 1990s, and early 2000s, when a pro-opioid movement in the medical pain community encouraged doctors to prescribe opioids more liberally and reassured them, based on false evidence, that the risk of becoming addicted to prescription opioids among patients being treated for pain was less than 1 percent[46] (see chapter 4). More recent studies reveal that as many as 56 percent of patients receiving long-term prescription opioid painkillers for low back pain, for example, progress to addictive opioid use, including patients with no prior history of addiction.[47]

The gateway hypothesis of addiction posits that using cigarettes and alcohol, which are legal drugs, leads to experimentation with other, "harder" drugs, like cocaine and heroin. Whether this progression is due simply to opportunity costs and ease of access,[48] or to some more fundamental biological mechanism based on the chemical composition of the drug itself,[49] is still being debated.

In today's world easy access to "harder" drugs through a doctor's prescription has turned the gateway hypothesis on its head. For increasing numbers of people, especially young people, prescription drugs are the first exposure to addictive substances and the first stepping-stone to future addictive use. My patient Justin's story provides an example of how a potent and addictive drug prescribed by a doctor can become a gateway to addiction.

Vicodin: A Gateway Drug

Justin had none of the classic risk factors of nature or nurture that we typically associate with increased risk of addiction. The only child of educated upper-middle-class Jewish parents, neither of whom (unlike Jim's parents) smoked, drank, or used drugs, and with no family history of addiction, he seemed at average risk. (A prevailing misconception is that Jewish people are at lower risk than other ethnic groups for substance use disorders. As told so well by Rabbi Shais Taub in the introduction of his excellent book *God of Our Understanding: Jewish Spirituality and Recovery from Addiction*, there are no data to support this stereotype.)[50]

Justin's childhood was also without trauma. His parents were loving, kind, and devoted to his well-being. He was in good physical health. Sometimes he was teased about his weight—he'd always been pudgy—but he never felt bullied. He had friends. He was neither impulsive nor prone to excessive emotionality. If anything his emotional expressions were muted. He was smart and schoolwork came easily to him. He especially liked science. He fondly remembers dissecting a cow's eye, and mixing cornstarch and water to make "oobleck," in the fourth grade. Anything having to do with computers was always of interest, in particular building computers and playing video games. He grew up in his parents' single-family home in a white middle-class suburb of San Francisco.

The risk factor that Justin encountered, contributing to his later development of addiction, had everything to do with neighborhood, and not neighborhood in the strict sense of geography, but neighborhood in the sense of context, culture, and technology. Justin, like many teens today, especially compared with previous generations, had early exposure to scheduled drugs (opioids) through a doctor's prescription, thereby developing a "taste" for them, followed by virtually unlimited access to drugs through peers at school and on the Internet.

During his sophomore year in high school, Justin went to the dentist to get his wisdom teeth removed. He lay back in the dentist's chair, the bright white lights slowly fading into blackness as he lost consciousness from the concoction of drugs the dentist had given him. When he awoke, it took him a moment to realize where he was. He heard the high-pitched whine of the drill and smelled the pungent odor of burnt enamel, and then he remembered: wisdom teeth. Despite his mouth being pulled apart by several sets of hands and a metal drill spinning near his flesh, he felt good—incredibly good, like no kind of good he could remember ever having felt before. He soon floated back into unconsciousness.

In the waiting room after the procedure was over and the drugs had mostly worn off, Justin felt nauseated, and his mouth was sore. Through a residual haze of the drugs' effect, he saw the dentist write out a prescription for Vicodin for pain relief. The dentist explained that Justin should take one pill every four to eight hours as needed for pain.

Once Justin and his mother arrived home, he took one pill and put the rest on his bedside table. He immediately felt relief from the pain in his mouth—and something else—an echo of that good feeling, that better-than-normal-for-him feeling. He lay in bed and again drifted off to sleep.

In the days that followed, Justin took one Vicodin every four hours. On the surface of things, his life had returned to normal. He was back at school, going through the motions of being an average high school student at the average California public high school in the mid-2000s. But inside, under the influence of Vicodin, he felt energized, worry free, and completely at ease with himself. He recalled the man who had visited their third-grade classroom to talk to them about the dangers of drugs and alcohol—part of the DARE project.* The man had told them that people took drugs to alter mood, to "feel good." Justin knew the man had meant it as a warning, but thinking about it now, the idea sounded like pure genius.

Justin began doubling up on the Vicodin, seeking to maintain the good feelings that had started to wear off with repeated use. When he ran out of his prescription, he asked his mother to take him back to the dentist to get more, telling her he still had pain. (His pain was mild and tolerable. What he was really looking for was a way to extend that sense of well-being that Vicodin provided.) His mother took him back to see the dentist, and the dentist readily prescribed Justin another month's supply. It surprised Justin how easy it was to get a refill and that no one questioned his motives.

An Epidemic of Overprescribing

The prescription drug epidemic is first and foremost an epidemic of overprescribing. Potions and elixirs have always been part of a doctor's trade, but today the extent to which doctors rely on prescription drugs, especially scheduled drugs, to treat their patients for even routine, non-life-threatening medical conditions is unprecedented.

In 2012, some 493,000 individuals aged 12 or older misused a prescription drug for the first time within the past twelve months,[35] an average of 1,350 initiatives per day. Of those who became addicted to

---

*The unintended consequences of drug use education are salient here. Drug Abuse Resistance Education (DARE) was a school-based prevention program, adopted throughout the United States in the late 1990s and early 2000s, in which police officers provided information on the dangers of drug use to students in the classroom. In retrospect, DARE was ineffective at preventing or even delaying drug use, and in some cases it may even have promoted use, as exemplified by Justin's experience. DARE illustrates the broader challenge of using didactic and mass media educational campaigns to target drug use.

any drug in the previous year, a quarter started out using a prescription medication: 17 percent began with opioid pain relievers, 5 percent with sedative-hypnotics, and 4 percent with stimulants.[35] Prescription drugs now rank fourth among the most-misused substances in America, behind alcohol, tobacco, and marijuana; and they rank second among teens.

Teens are especially vulnerable to the increased access to prescription drugs. Adolescence is a time when the rapidly growing brain is more plastic, and therefore more vulnerable on a neurological level, to potentially irreversible brain changes caused by chronic drug exposure.[51, 52] Teens are more vulnerable to social contagion pressures to experiment with drugs. Also, most importantly, ready access to heroin and methamphetamine equivalents in pill form has blurred the lines between soft and hard drugs for today's youth.

When the second refill ran out, Justin was reluctant to ask for more. But despite daily use for more than a month, he didn't suffer any acute physical opioid withdrawal. However, that single exposure to opioid painkillers set him on a new course. He began experimenting with a variety of prescription pharmaceuticals, which was normative among his peers, who generally viewed prescription pills as safer than illegal drugs. He obtained all his pills from school friends, mostly for free, but sometimes for cash. His friends got pills from a combination of doctors, relatives, and drug dealers. Justin liked prescription opioid painkillers best of all.

Justin ingested drugs almost exclusively during school hours, so by the time he went home, the effects had worn off and his parents didn't notice. Amazingly, neither did his teachers. One day in the middle of class, Justin took SOMA, a potent muscle relaxant. As he began to feel its effects, he had an uncontrollable desire to stretch out and extend his muscles. Sitting at the back of the class, he began gyrating in circles with his upper body, leaning far over his desk, to the right, then the left, then backward, almost sliding off his chair in the process. As he remembers it, no one noticed, or at least no one commented. Either way, it's disconcerting to think such behavior can go unremarked.

Justin was slated to graduate from high school in 2006, but he failed an English class his senior year, and never got around to making it up. Instead he spent the next couple of years hanging out with friends and using drugs, mostly cannabis, alcohol, and whatever pills they could easily get from one another. He took a couple of classes at the community college, but didn't really apply himself. He finally took and passed his GED in 2009.

His parents weren't sure what to make of his desultory lifestyle in those years after high school. Justin believes they knew about the marijuana, which they were okay with because his dad had used pot on weekends in his youth; but they were oblivious to Justin's use of other drugs and to the extent of the pot use, and they were unaware that the pot Justin smoked was much more potent than anything his dad had access to in the 1970s.

It's easy in retrospect to condemn parents who seem not to notice that their kids are using drugs, but I've met too many caring parents over the years to stand in judgment. Kids using drugs go to great lengths to conceal their use, and even watchful parents can miss the signs.

Cyberpharmacies

After high school, Justin gradually lost contact with his drug-sourcing high school friends and thereby lost a ready supply of pot and pills. Being risk-averse by nature, he was reluctant to seek out drug dealers, try to get drugs from doctors by feigning illness (doctor shop), or do anything else overtly illegal to get drugs. Instead, he discovered a new source that was convenient, cheap, and didn't require him to leave the safety and comfort of his own home: the Internet.

Justin's parents were both at work, and though he was supposed to be spending time online looking at courses to enroll in the local community college, or looking for a job, he was instead typing "Vicodin," still his drug of choice, into Google. That query pulled up links for online pharmaceutical companies. He clicked on Top Ten Meds Online, which looked like a legitimate pharmaceutical company, but just to be sure, he googled it on SafeorScam.com, an online resource that would tell him whether this site was some kind of sting operation or scam. It checked out, so he went back and searched for Vicodin. None was available. Next, he typed in "opioids" and found codeine as a cough medicine. He put it in his cart. He typed in "tranquilizer/hypnotic" and put Valium and Xanax in his cart. Just before heading to checkout, he added the dissociative anesthetic ketamine. He entered his credit card information and clicked the purchase button. Within the week, his "medications" were shipped to his house, delivered by FedEx, no prescription required.

Law enforcement agencies first became aware of online pharmacies selling controlled substances without a prescription in the mid-1990s, coinciding with reports on the rapid increase in prescription opioid abuse and misuse and prescription opioid–related overdoses, especially among young people. These websites conduct business in the United States in direct violation of the United States Controlled Substance Act (CSA).

Despite operating in violation of the CSA, websites that sell controlled medications without a prescription are difficult for law enforcement to monitor or prosecute. As described in the article by Forman and coauthors, "The Internet as a Source of Drugs of Abuse," the web page for such a site may be physically located in Uzbekistan, the business address in Mexico City, money generated from purchases deposited in a bank in the Cayman Islands, the drugs themselves shipped from India, while the owner of the site is living in Florida. Law enforcement from multiple countries would have to collaborate to enforce and prosecute the owner of a single site, and the entire operation can be dismantled, erased, and reestablished elsewhere in a single day.[53] Furthermore, marketing techniques used by the sites make it difficult to find them. Some of these no-prescription online sites camouflage themselves as something other than a drug-selling site. One such site went by the name "Christian Site for the Whole Family," with links to "bible study group" and "Easter Drugs Sale: Buy Codeine without a Prescription."[53]

The international nature of the drug trade today gives the old opium wars, as commented on by Walsh, a new twist, wherein cyberpharmacists are drug dealers for the modern age.[54] Support for this claim comes from a report out of Columbia University, which gathered data showing that 11 percent of the prescriptions filled in 2006 by traditional (brick and mortar) pharmacies were for controlled (scheduled) substances, whereas 95 percent of the prescriptions filled by online pharmacies in the same year were for controlled substances.[55]

The Internet is not merely a passive portal for controlled prescription drugs. Once Justin, for example, has purchased drugs online, the site remembers him and may send unsolicited e-mails alerting him to new products or special deals. This aspect makes it especially difficult for addicted individuals to stop using drugs. Short of changing his e-mail address or utilizing filtering software, Justin cannot avoid being found and targeted once again for drug use by Internet sellers.

Initially Justin looked only for prescription drugs through online pharmacies, but gradually he became interested in new and experimental drugs in the pharmaceutical pipeline, often sold as "research chemicals." He learned about new drugs by spending time on the website Pipemania.com, a splinter group of Lifetheuniverseandeverything .com. Pipemania, one of many Internet communities like it, is a forum where users talk about what drugs they are using and what those drugs feel like, including lots of newly synthesized drugs and newer drug combinations. People using these sites refer to themselves as "researchers" and to their drug use experiences as "research findings."

Examples of newer synthetic drugs include Methoxetamine, or MXE, an analog of the drug ketamine, labeled as a "research chemical product" and taken for its hallucinogenic and dissociative effects. Purple Drank, or Lean, another popular new mixture consumed primarily by young people, combines Sprite, Jolly Ranchers, and codeine (an opioid). If prescription codeine is unavailable, DM (dextromethorphan) cough syrup is often substituted.

The buying and selling of illegal drugs, outside of online pharmacies, occurs primarily in the "deep web," a term used to refer to a clandestine part of the network where online activity can be kept anonymous. Most of these drug-selling underground sites use Bitcoin as their only currency, providing customers with anonymous access to drugs from all over the world, without even a pretense at legality. One such site, now dismantled, was Silk Road, allegedly operated by 30-year-old Ross W. Ulbricht, who went by the pseudonym Dread Pirate Roberts, a character from the movie *The Princess Bride*. Mr. Ulbricht was recently convicted of narcotics trafficking, computer hacking, and money laundering.

Heroin—the New Vicodin

In 2012, despite engaging in daily, now mostly solitary, drug use, Justin attended community college and got a job at Oracle in the shipping department. With his new job, he was suddenly in possession of cash, and much more than he had become accustomed to with his parents' allowance. One night in the summer of that year, he went to a small get-together at a friend's house, where he met someone whose brother knew a heroin dealer. Justin had never tried heroin before; he had always shied away from illegal so-called street drugs and from drug dealers. But he was curious, and eager to use opioids, which were increasingly difficult to obtain online in any form. Through friends he met Sean, the man who would become his heroin dealer, his business partner, and his housemate. Justin bought a gram of heroin, telling himself it was no big deal; it was just an experiment, and he could handle it.

Heroin was originally synthesized in 1874 by C. R. Alder Wright, an English chemist working at St. Mary's Hospital Medical School in London. Wright added two acetyl groups to morphine to form di-acetylated morphine, which was largely forgotten until twenty-three years later, when it was independently synthesized by Felix Hoffmann in Germany. Hoffmann, working at what is today the Bayer Group's Pharmaceutical Division, was instructed to find a less addictive alternative to morphine. Di-acetylated morphine was marketed by Bayer alongside aspirin from 1898 to 1910 as a nonaddictive morphine substitute and cough suppressant, as well as a cure for morphine addiction. Bayer named di-acetylated morphine "heroin," based on the German "heroisch," which means "heroic" or "strong." Strong it certainly was. By the early 1900s an epidemic of heroin addiction raged in the United States, prompting passage of the Harrison Narcotic Act of 1914 to control the sale and distribution of heroin and other opioids. Today in the United States, heroin is considered a schedule I drug, meaning it is considered highly addictive and is not approved for any medical purpose.

Justin intended to use his heroin sparingly, just now and then. Instead he used it daily for two months, not stopping till he had run through the entire $1,600 he had earned and saved from his job at Oracle. He lost his job and quit school, unable to meet the demands of either. Then he went into acute heroin withdrawal. He remembers heroin withdrawal as "the most horrible feeling in the world, like you're gonna die." Elaborating further, "I wouldn't wish it on anyone, not my worst enemy."

The number of Americans aged 12 and older who used heroin in the past month rose from 281,000 to 335,000 between 2011 and 2013, a significant increase from the 166,000 using heroin in 2002.[56] According to the Centers for Disease Control and Prevention, heroin-related overdose deaths also rose in that time frame, with a 39 percent increase between 2012 and 2013 alone. The majority of new heroin users cite prescription opioids as their first exposure to opioids,[57] a clear generational shift. In the 1960s, 80 percent of opioid users reported that their first exposure to opioids was in the form of heroin. In the 2000s, 75 percent of opioid users reported that their first exposure to opioids was in the form of prescription painkillers.[58] Increases in heroin use have been driven mostly by 18–25 year olds.

Justin went to Sean and told him he was out of money, but desperate for heroin. Sean offered Justin an arrangement in which Justin would work for Sean, and in exchange, get cheap access to heroin for his services. Sean wanted Justin to sell for him, but Justin wasn't willing. As an alternative, Sean offered that Justin could work in "his lab," an offer which Justin accepted.

For the next nine months, Justin spent most of his time at Sean's house, running Sean's lab. Sean lived in a rundown house in a rundown neighborhood in East Oakland, a place with hardly any furniture besides a TV, a plastic kitchen table with plastic chairs, and a couple of worn mattresses. Justin had dropped out of school, unable to keep up with his courses while strung out on heroin. He told his parents he was "staying with a friend," and he returned home every two or three days for a visit, just to reassure them all was well.

On a typical day during those nine months between the summer of 2012, when Justin first tried heroin, and spring of 2013, when he would first attempt to quit, Sean and Justin would wake up around one in the afternoon and share a light breakfast. This breakfast did not consist of food; it consisted of heroin. They both preferred snorting to injecting. They lined the heroin up on a smooth, clean surface and passed it between them till they were sated, just as if they were passing a basket of rolls. Sometimes they "chased the dragon," a way of ingesting heroin that requires putting the heroin on a bit of tin foil, putting a source of heat—a match or a lighter—below the foil, and inhaling the vaporized powder. The term "chasing the dragon" refers to the plume of smoke that rises up off the foil, like a mythical dragon's tail, as well as the high that addicted persons seek, as elusive as the mythical creature whose name it bears.

Justin recalls that he was never hungry when he was using heroin. In fact, he didn't want anything. He didn't want to eat, read, bathe, exercise, watch TV, or even play his beloved video games. He was living in a "dump" with no furniture, no food in the refrigerator, no family, no job, and no prospects for the future, and despite the ever-present threat of legal consequences from dealing in illegal drugs, he felt "complete."

He spent his days cooking heroin from morphine, and when the stink of the chemicals made his eyes burn, he joined Sean on the porch. Every hour or two they snorted heroin. "Because we were distributors, we didn't even wait till we were feeling sick to use. We'd use to get even higher than we already were."

The First Step to Recovery

One day in the spring of 2013, Justin was sitting in Sean's house filling balloon bags of heroin for later sale, when he realized that he had been using heroin daily for exactly nine months. "I was thinking in my head, 'Wow, it's been almost a year. If I let this year go by, it's going to be five years, ten years, maybe my whole life.'" At that moment he decided to quit. He also recognized that he would not be able to act on his decision without help, primarily due to the physiologic withdrawal associated with stopping opioids.

Again he turned to the Internet. While the latest batch of heroin was still cooking in the oven, Justin looked up treatment for heroin addiction on his laptop. He found a website for BAART (Bay Area Addiction Research and Treatment), a methadone maintenance treatment clinic in Oakland, and immediately set up an appointment. (For a discussion of methadone and Suboxone, opioid agonist treatments for opioid addiction, see chapter 5). Justin recalls that BAART required their clients to be in active withdrawal when initiating methadone, so he stopped using in the hours before his appointment and was plenty sick when he went in and received his first dose of methadone.

Justin also decided to tell his parents. He realized he'd have to be living at home again, and traveling every morning to Oakland to get his methadone dose, and there was all the paperwork he needed to fill out. There was no way he could hide it from them any longer.

The same day he started on methadone, Justin told his parents that heroin was something he'd always wanted to try and thought he could handle. He said he'd been sucked in, and he blamed no one but himself. He knew his parents felt guilty anyway, as if they had failed him. Justin almost cried remembering their conversation. "They were very supportive," he said. "They've always been very supportive."

Justin did well on methadone. He enrolled at the community college again, made new nonusing friends, and joined a study group. When he did relapse six months after being in the BAART program, he relapsed hard—which is common—and was smoking crack at the same time he was using heroin. He dropped out of the methadone program at BAART, but bought methadone on the street to ease his comedowns. For months he managed to use crack and heroin on the weekends and methadone to get through his classes during the week. One day, unable to reach his methadone source, he started to go into withdrawal. "I realized 'I'm at the whim of my dealer.'" He bought some Suboxone, a medication with similarities to methadone, also used to treat opioid addiction, from a friend, and used that the same way he had used methadone, that is, to tide him over when he couldn't get heroin.

But Justin was getting tired. Tired of chasing down heroin, methadone, and Suboxone. Tired of feeling anxious and sick, wondering if he'd have enough drug to keep going. Tired of lying and living the double life—pretending, as he says, "to be sober, but having this second actual life where you're keeping secrets from everybody, lying, and having to keep track of all the lies. It's all just so hard to keep up."

Again he looked on the Internet, this time for someone to prescribe Suboxone, which is how he found me. When he told me his story, I agreed that Suboxone made sense, given the severity of his opioid addiction. But Suboxone treatment requires close monitoring, including regular clinic visits and urine toxicology screens to test for the presence of other drugs. If other drugs are detected, I explained, ongoing Suboxone treatment might be compromised. I also encouraged him to seek some kind of psychosocial intervention to treat his addiction as well.

Justin agreed to Suboxone treatment and monitoring and to a Narcotics Anonymous (NA) meeting. Unlike Jim, he did not find twelve-step groups helpful; they just weren't for him. He quit going after a few weeks. But Justin came to appointments regularly and never tested positive for other drugs, except for a couple of small slipups with benzodiazepines, the most recent when, while cleaning his room, he came across an old stash of Valium pressed between his bed and the wall. He took the Valium for sleep for the next several weeks, then stopped. He felt guilty about it. A year later, he is still doing well.

A Different Kind of Dragon

Justin ascribes his year of recovery from addiction to Suboxone, his relationship with his parents, and interactive role-playing tabletop games. "Suboxone stops the cravings and I can feel normal. I don't lie anymore. Role-playing games help by giving me the escape and excitement that I would usually get from that whole street life."

Today, Justin spends most of his weekdays studying. On the weekends, he spends some time on the computer, but he no longer visits online pharmacies or spends nearly the amount of time he used to playing video games. Instead, with some sweet irony, he is much more likely to be on a site called Penandpaper.com. There he is able to interact with other players of so-called tabletop, or role-player games. Tabletop games simulate the quest story lines so popular among video gamers, but without the video. There is often an online version of the role-player games, but Justin much prefers the face-to-face version. He claims the story is richer that way.

On a typical Saturday, Justin's five tabletop teammates, now a stable crew he meets with on a regular basis for gaming, come to his house around eleven o'clock to spend the day playing. Collaborative storytelling is the essence of the game. They sit around a table, sometimes for as long as eight hours at a time, and together describe the world their characters will inhabit and what will happen to them in that world. Sometimes they may even act out a scene or engage in a small role-play, as if creating theater, though none of them would ever describe themselves as actors.

They are currently playing ShadowRun, set in a futuristic world populated by magical beings and cyborgs. Justin's character is an Ork, a troll-like creature with robotic enhancements and cybernetic abilities named "J-Rez." Their latest story line bears an uncanny resemblance to Justin's own life—and it can be read as the narrative of Justin's alter ego.

J-Rez has just heard from his female crime boss that his next mission is to travel to Seattle to obtain a new synthetic drug called Novacoke. In Seattle, J-Rez meets up with the other members of the organized crime ring, and together they venture into a high-crime neighborhood to deliver a package of research chemicals needed to make Novacoke. In exchange, they get a sample of the drug to take back to their boss. However, right after getting the package they came for, they are nearly killed by a detonated bomb, saved only by J-Rez's robotic enhancements. The team then combs the neighborhood and, through diligent detective work, including deciphering a tattoo, identifies their would-be killer—a man who has eluded them because he has the ability to turn into a dragon. J-Rez and his gang embark on their next assignment: chasing the dragon.

Justin continues to chase mythical creatures, but for now, not through the medium of addictive drugs.

The Gateway Now a Runway

Young people today don't just experiment with cigarettes, alcohol, and marijuana. They try everything, especially if it comes in the form of a pill. They even try chemicals newly synthesized in a laboratory without any idea of what these chemicals might do to them. They obtain these drugs from friends at school, from the Internet, from their own home chemistry kits. The gateway, in other words, has become a runway, telescoping the progression from recreational to addictive use. That first prescription for opioids, stimulants, or sedatives is the boarding pass, in some cases, to a lifelong struggle with addiction.

3

Pain Is Dangerous, Difference Is Psychopathology
The Role of Illness Narratives

Let's return to the story of my patient Jim, whom we left in a Bay Area hospital being treated for a lower-back infection. Jim's doctors prescribed a dose of morphine as needed every four hours, a standard order for patients in the hospital struggling with severe pain and a time-saver for nurses and doctors, allowing the nurse to administer pain relievers without having to call the doctor back every time. For some patients, such an order is compassionate care. For others, like Jim, that kind of order is poison.

By the second time the nurse came around with the morphine, Jim knew what was coming, and he was already feeling the high just anticipating it. He rested his head back on the pillow, proffered his left arm with the percutaneous intravenous line ready and, taking a deep breath, thought, "Now I'm going to feel real good, and I don't have to be embarrassed about it, because I'm a patient, and these are doctors giving me this drug."

Of central importance here is the way Jim's new identity as a patient encouraged him to create an autobiographical narrative that justified his use of pain meds.

Autobiographical narratives are the stories we tell about our lives, and they are as fundamental to human existence as breathing. Our life stories connect us to others, organize experience, and shape time. Autobiographical narratives are deeply influenced by the prevailing culture—religious affiliation, ethnic background, contemporaneous historical events. Culture not only provides the frame of reference in which life narratives are told but also influences the perception and memory of the experiences themselves. Jerome Bruner, in an essay entitled "Life as Narrative," says that "the culturally shaped cognitive and linguistic processes that guide the self-telling of life narratives achieve the power to structure perceptual experience, to organize memory, to segment and purpose-build the very 'events' of a life. In the end, we become the autobiographical narratives by which we 'tell about' our lives" (694).[59] Culture shapes narrative, and narrative shapes experience.

As a hospitalized patient in pain, Jim could experience the high of morphine without the accompanying guilt and shame that had contaminated his pleasure in drinking during the latter years of his alcohol addiction. Jim's new narrative was possible because of new cultural norms concerning the nature and meaning of pain. Today, the experience of pain in any form is fraught with danger, in large part because pain, so the thinking goes, puts the individual at risk to experience future pain.

Pain Is Dangerous

For millennia, we have understood pain in our lives to serve at least two useful functions. First, pain is a warning system: what to avoid and what not. Second, pain is an opportunity for spiritual growth: "What doesn't kill you makes you stronger," "After darkness comes the dawn," etc. Today, pain is little valued for these reasons. Instead, modern American culture regards pain as anathema, to be avoided at all cost. This new way of looking at pain arises from the belief that pain can cause permanent neurological damage that lays the foundation for future pain. This new conception holds true for both mental and physical pain, and it has been a major contributor to the prescription drug epidemic.

Mental Pain as a Psychic Scar

Our culture is steeped in the idea that psychological trauma creates a psychic wound that is the source of future suffering. The classic example of this is post-traumatic stress disorder, which holds that any kind of trauma can lead to future symptoms of anxiety, disturbing memories, abnormal autonomic function, extreme and maladaptive avoidant behavior, and so on. The Canadian philosopher Ian Hacking writes about the "traumatization of experience, in other words, the conceptualization of the past event as a painful scar."[60]

The origin of this idea dates back at least to Freud, whose groundbreaking psychoanalytic contribution (early 1900s) was the idea that early childhood experiences can influence behavior in later life. Our awareness of these early experiences and their impact on our emotions and behaviors can occur outside of conscious awareness. Unconscious childhood trauma is in turn the root of many forms of psychopathology. The idea that an experience in one's past can have a lasting psychological and often unconscious effect on one's behavior in the present is one that we practically take for granted today, but it was a profoundly radical idea, one that changed the way twentieth-century Western peoples understood their lives.

Chronic Pain and Centralized Pain Syndromes

The role of physical pain has likewise undergone a similar transformation. Two hundred years ago, physical pain was viewed by most physicians as a desirable component of the healing process.[61] Pain was believed to be especially salutary during surgery, by invigorating cardiovascular function and bolstering the immune response. By the mid-1850s, improved treatments for pain, such as morphine and the hollow-needle syringe used to administer it, invented by Alexander Wood in 1855, contributed to changing views about treatment. With a viable alternative for treating pain, more doctors began advocating for the use of opioid painkillers.[61] By the 1950s, pain as its own discipline was born within the medical profession, driven by refined technology that allowed for opioids to be readily synthesized in the laboratory and by an efficient pharmaceutical industry eager to sell them. This new industry, more than any other factor, legitimized the treatment of pain as a medical subspecialty unto itself, requiring its own training and board certification.

Today, pain is considered an almost intolerable sensation for patients to endure. Doctors are expected not just to lessen pain, but to eliminate it altogether. The pressure to treat pain has become so overwhelming that doctors who leave pain untreated are not just demonstrating poor clinical skills; they are viewed as morally compromised. They are also legally liable for malpractice.

The concept of pain as a long-term condition that can occur independently of illness or injury is also very much a late-twentieth-century phenomenon. Prior to 1900, pain was a response to acute illness or injury, and there was as yet no concept of chronic (long-lasting) pain. It is now commonly accepted within medicine that a patient can experience physical pain that lasts months, even years, in the absence of any disease process or recognizable physical injury. Indeed, the list of different types of chronic pain syndrome seems to be growing every day, including complex regional pain syndrome, failed back syndrome, fibromyalgia, interstitial cystitis, myofascial pain syndrome, postvasectomy pain, vulvodynia, pelvic pain syndrome—and on and on.

Today it is entirely commonplace to see a young, otherwise healthy individual with no obvious injury or disease present to a medical doctor seeking help for "corpedynia," "corpe" for body and "dynia" for pain— full-body pain. These patients describe experiencing pain from the tips of their toes to the ends of their eyelashes. They undergo a full medical workup to rule out recognizable causes of pain. Once those have been eliminated, the patients are not carted off to the psychiatrist, as they might have been prior to 1950. Instead they are given a variant diagnosis of "chronic pain," such as fibromyalgia.

As with psychological injury, physical pain, if not treated immediately, is also believed to have the potential to contribute to future pain. This phenomenon is known as "central sensitization," and pain researchers talk about "pain hypersensitivity . . . and secondary changes in brain activity that can be detected by electrophysiological or imaging techniques."[62] Pain researchers' speculations that once the individual experiences pain, the brain can be sensitized for future pain (making physical pain not just a source of immediate suffering but also a potential source of future suffering), created yet additional urgency to treat pain immediately and completely.

We have arrived at a new, much lower threshold of tolerance for how much pain is too much pain for an individual to suffer. Ironically, as our lives have become progressively more comfortable, with modernization, increased leisure time, and decreased threat of illness and injury, we have become less and less able to tolerate any kind of pain. For patients seeking treatment for physical and mental pain, these new norms have contributed to increased prescribing and consumption of potentially addictive prescription drugs.

Difference Is Psychopathology

Another contemporary illness narrative that has contributed to the prescription drug epidemic, is one in which individual differences in emotionality, cognition, and temperament are increasingly defined as illness. When human differences are defined as illness, it naturally follows that medical treatment is necessary to eliminate those differences. This idea is fueled by our contemporary view of mental disorders, in which thoughts, feelings, and actions are nothing more than neurons firing in a chemical soup. Changing brain chemistry becomes the new way to normalize differences.

The case of my patient Karen illustrates the ways in which identifying and labeling innate differences as a form of brain pathology can lead, over time, to medicating those differences with potentially addictive prescription medications that can ultimately lead to addiction. Karen's story is not meant to suggest that every person who is diagnosed with mental illness and treated with a scheduled drug has been misdiagnosed or will inevitably fall prey to addiction. Indeed, some people are well served by giving their innate differences a name and providing "treatment" in the form of medication or otherwise. Karen's story is merely a cautionary tale.

Born in the mid-1980s to loving, well-heeled parents, Karen was a healthy, happy child, with no early signs or symptoms of illness, mental or otherwise. Furthermore, her parents remember her as a kind and gregarious child who excelled at sports. In elementary school, she made friends easily, and with her prowess at ball sports and her easygoing nature, she was a leader on the playground. However, she demonstrated difficulty with reading comprehension and memory tasks compared to her peers. The school psychologist diagnosed her with a nonspecific "learning disability." Once the diagnosis had been made, Karen's parents and the school mobilized to provide Karen with additional support to overcome her disability. She got help from tutors, education experts and psychologists, and with their support, her reading improved.

In middle school Karen continued to struggle with academics, but on the basketball court, her ability to learn was intact. In high school she became a top basketball player and was recruited by several colleges to play at the collegiate level. She decided to forgo playing basketball in college, however, to focus on academics, consistent with the more conservative traditions of her family. Karen arrived at college in 2005 with high expectations but without the support structure she was used to. The classes were huge, the material more challenging, and she had no more tutors to help her. She was faced with unprecedented amounts of free time that she wasn't sure how to organize. She struggled to work efficiently, and reading was still a chore.

Despite these early challenges, Karen was able to do moderately well in her college classes in her first couple of years. But she was ambitious, and in her junior year she decided to major in both art history and graphic design. She was required to increase the number of classes she was taking and with the added pressure, was quickly overwhelmed. She saw some of her peers taking more classes and doing well, and she wondered why she couldn't do the same.

Two of Karen's best friends had been diagnosed with attention deficit disorder (ADD)—similar to attention deficit hyperactivity disorder (ADHD) but without the high energy component—and were taking stimulant medication (for example, Adderall or Ritalin). Karen wondered if ADD might be a possible explanation for her inability to excel with the increased course load. She decided to see a doctor and get tested.

She met with a psychiatrist, answered a series of questions dating back to childhood—questions on her ability to concentrate, sit still, get organized, accomplish tasks. Based on one visit, the doctor diagnosed ADD and wrote Karen a prescription for Adderall extended release (XR) formulation 15 mg daily, as well as Adderall immediate release (IR) 10 mg daily.

Adderall is an FDA schedule II drug, which means that, although it has been shown to have medical benefit, it also has a high potential for misuse and addiction. It is molecularly similar to the street drug methamphetamine, also known as "ice" or "crank." Adderall has been used for decades as a performance enhancing drug in the military, but not until the 1980s was it common practice to prescribe Adderall and other stimulants for the treatment of attention deficit disorder, including prescribing it to children and adolescents. The total numbers of prescriptions for stimulants dispensed by US pharmacies between 1991 and 2010 increased tenfold.[63] Prescriptions for stimulants among school age children (5–18 years) nearly tripled between 1990 and 1995 alone.[64]

When Karen took Adderall, she could sit in a chair for hours at a time, at home or at the library, studying, and she retained the material better. She understood her response as validation of her diagnosis of ADD. This kind of backward logic prevails in the mental health care field: if the medicine makes you feel better, then your diagnosis must be whatever the medicine was meant to treat. We know, however, that stimulants will make almost anyone better able to focus, concentrate, and perform certain types of tasks, even in the absence of a cognitive disorder. Likewise, benzodiazepines (Xanax) help people relax in the absence of anxiety, sedatives (Ambien) induce sleep in the absence of insomnia, and opioids (Vicodin) enhance subjective well-being in the absence of pain.

We are all born with inherent mental and physical differences. What is striking in our culture today is how readily those differences are labeled as illness and treated with a pill. From early childhood onward, Karen's learning differences were framed as brain pathology. Her relative lack of aptitude for reading was called a learning disability, and her struggles in college diagnosed as attention deficit disorder. This is not to invalidate Karen's relative difficulties with reading or other academic pursuits. But in embracing these differences as "disabilities" or "disorders," our culture is implicitly rejecting alternative narratives, for example, that human differences in temperament and ability are valuable and should be celebrated and that human differences should be understood in terms of sociological, existential, and even spiritual etiologies, rather than purely biological ones.

An experienced psychologist who treats college and graduate students at a university student mental health clinic described it this way: "What I frequently see in my 20- to 30-something patients is they come to therapy self-identifying with mental health disorders that were diagnosed in adolescence. They take meds and are fearful that the stress of their lives will trigger their 'illness.' Almost always the flares of 'illness' are triggered by difficult life events, but the go-to intervention that they always turn to is an adjustment to the medication."

In *The Myth of Mental Illness*, Thomas Szasz famously declared that mental illness does not exist because there are no specific anatomical or molecular markers that define it.[65] Mental illness, according to Szasz, is merely a means by which "the therapeutic state" exerts social control on its citizens, for example, by enforced temporary hospitalization of the mentally ill. I do not agree with Szasz that mental illness does not exist; the absence of biological markers is not the absence of disease. As Clarke describes in a critique of Szasz,[66] for many years we did not know what caused malaria, until certain advances in molecular science made its discovery possible. Yet we knew the disease of malaria when we saw it. Likewise the patient with schizophrenia, psychotic mania, severe obsessive compulsive disorder, etc., is struggling with a brain disease, even if we can't necessarily measure it or see it under a microscope. But Szasz's point that we risk coercing conformity by labeling all deviant behavior as mental illness is relevant here. A prime historical example is homosexuality, which was considered a mental illness as recently 1973.[67]

Today, our definition of mental illness subsumes not only deviancy but even subtle differences between us. It has become a way to understand not only failure to conform but also failure to excel. Now even the average underachiever and the quirky recluse risk a diagnosis of mental illness. For some individuals, receiving a diagnosis of a mental illness is no doubt helpful, giving them access to resources they might otherwise not have had and providing them with a framework to understand their differences, without which they might have felt stigmatized and ashamed. What concerns me is the leap between diagnosing differences and treating differences with a pill, especially when that pill carries with it the risk of addiction.

Doctors are of course complicit in this process, particularly psychiatrists, who over the last thirty years have increasingly turned to psychoactive drugs to manage their patients' emotional distress, psychiatric symptoms, or life crises, leaving the business of psychotherapy to others.[68] Why have psychiatrists largely abandoned their roots in psychoanalysis and other forms of talk therapy in favor of the magic of the pill? They have done so in part because they have become true believers in the reductionistic, biologized view of human behavior (neurons firing in a chemical soup). Financial incentives for doctors to prescribe pills have also contributed to this trend (see chapter 8).

This paradigm shift has created an entire generation of young people, most notably the millennials (1980–2000), who have embraced the promise of better living through chemistry. From 1998 to 2008, the percentage of Americans who took at least one prescription drug in the past month increased from 44 percent to 48 percent. The use of two or more drugs increased from 25 percent to 31 percent. The use of five or more drugs increased from 6 percent to 11 percent. In 2007, one of every five American children and nine out of ten older Americans (age 60 and older) reported using at least one prescription drug in the past month. The most commonly used types of drug are central nervous system stimulants for adolescents and antidepressants for middle-aged adults. In the United States, spending for prescription drugs was $234.1 billion in 2008, more than double the amount spent in 1999.[69]

Many of today's youth think nothing of taking Adderall (a stimulant) in the mornings to get themselves going, Vicodin (an opioid painkiller) after lunch to treat a sport's injury, "medical" marijuana in the evening to relax, and Xanax (a benzodiazepine) at night to put themselves to sleep, all prescribed by a doctor. Getting the equivalent of those prescriptions from a friend, a family member, or even a drug dealer is not a very big stretch. Twenty-six percent of today's teens believe that prescription drugs are a good study aid.[70] Two-thirds of college seniors will be offered prescription stimulants for nonmedical use, and 31 percent will use a prescription stimulant for nonmedical use at least once during their college career.[71] The number of cases of prescription stimulant intoxication or misuse in adolescents rose 76 percent between 1998 and 2005.[72] Prescription drugs are now the second most-misused category of drug among adolescents, behind only marijuana.[73]

My young patients have candidly asked me, "What really is the difference between a medication you prescribe, and a drug I get from a friend or buy on the street to do the same thing?" I have responded with complex justifications involving legality and safety. But the real answer is, not very much. Sadly, the unintended consequence of being weaned on pharmaceuticals is a vicious and unprecedented scourge of addiction.

From Medicating an Illness to Feeding an Addiction

Karen began staying up late into the night doing work and was so productive with the Adderall that she was reluctant to waste her time sleeping when she could get so much done. She often didn't get to sleep till two in the morning. She stayed in on weekends to work on school projects, forgoing social activities with friends. Soon, nothing was as rewarding as working, and although her friends expressed dismay at her increasing reclusiveness, Karen was celebrated by her teachers for her productivity.

After graduating from college in 2009, Karen went to design school. Her dream was to be an interior decorator. She found a New York psychiatrist on Google who advertised expertise in treating ADD. Karen went to the doctor, paid for the visit in cash, and got a prescription for Adderall XR 20 mg daily and Adderall IR 20 mg daily. The psychiatrist did not ask for collateral information or prior records to verify diagnosis or dose. The session lasted less than fifteen minutes.

Furthermore, her new psychiatrist told her that Adderall IR could be taken on an "as needed" basis, that is to say, "whenever you're having symptoms." With this advice, Karen began taking the medication not only when she was having trouble studying or working but increasingly when she struggled with any kind of negative emotion—anxiety, sadness, frustration, boredom. The medicine lifted her mood and improved her energy—proof, she reasoned, that ADD was the cause of her distress.

Over the next two years, seeing the same doctor, Karen's dose gradually increased to Adderall XR 25 mg daily and Adderall IR 20 mg twice a day, more than double what she had started on in college. Her visits with the doctor were very short, sometimes no more than ten minutes. Karen never said much, except to emphasize how well she was doing and how much the Adderall was helping her function in the world.

However, Karen now reflects that, despite telling others she was thriving, in reality her life was beginning to fall apart. She was sleeping little, spending all her time working, barely seeing her friends, and no longer dating at all. She failed to show up for meetings and classes, always canceling at the last minute. She developed overwhelming anxiety in social situations, which she had never had before. She spent more and more time alone, in her apartment, nominally "doing work."

"Doing work became my excuse for doing Adderall. I had to be successful, and I needed the Adderall to do the work, not realizing I did better work when I didn't take the Adderall."

Studies show that stimulants like Adderall enhance memory and attention, but there is little or no research on their effects on abstract thought or creativity.[74] Indeed, there may be a trade-off between the ability to have laser focus to complete a specific task and the ability to let the mind wander, make new connections, and create something new.

Hanif Kureishi, writing in the *New York Times* in an essay called "The Art of Distraction," reflects:

> Sometimes things get done better when you're doing something else. If you're writing and you get stuck, and you then make tea, while waiting for the kettle to boil the chances are good ideas will occur to you. Seeing that a sentence has to have a particular shape can't be forced; you have to wait for your own judgment to inform you, and it usually does, in time. Some interruptions are worth having if they create a space for something to work in the fertile unconscious. Indeed, some distractions are more than useful; they might be more like realizations and can be as informative and multilayered as dreams. They might be where the excitement is.[75]

In early 2011, Karen's psychiatrist was out of town when Karen needed a refill. Desperate for her medications, she found a self-advertised

"ADD psychiatrist" on Google and went to see him. Karen knew what to say. It was easy to get this doctor to write her another prescription. Karen now had two psychiatrists filling the same prescription.

"I didn't feel I was doing anything wrong—getting the same prescription from two different doctors—which is really weird looking back on it. I told myself I needed the medication for an illness. I needed it to survive. But the truth was, I had started putting the drug above food and sleep and my own ethics."

In July 2011 Karen moved back to California to live with her parents and look for a job. The next three years of Karen's life were filled with lots of doctors, lots of Adderall prescriptions, and lots of juggling doctors to get those prescriptions. Her standard reported dosage to any doctor she visited was now Adderall XR 50 mg daily (*Physician's Desk Reference* maximum daily dose of Adderall XR is 20 mg), plus Adderall IR 20 mg twice daily. When a doctor balked at prescribing that much, Karen always agreed to start at a lower dose and then cajoled them into prescribing higher doses over time. For her the key to getting her doctors to increase the dose over time was to emphasize how functional she was with the medication, how nonfunctional without it, and how much she appreciated their help, none of which, from her perspective, was a lie. By now her evolving illness narrative had legs. That she was getting multiple prescriptions from multiple doctors and lying to them about lost prescriptions and lost bottles to get more of the drug represented a minor wrinkle in the larger fabric of the story she and her doctors had woven together over time: she had an illness, namely, ADD, and the Adderall was effective treatment for that illness.

By 2013, Karen had three different doctors prescribing Adderall at the same time, for a minimum daily consumption of Adderall XR 150 mg and Adderall IR 120 mg daily. Karen began stealing money from her parents because her insurance would only cover one prescription per month. She needed on average $1,200 per month just to be able to afford her prescriptions. She lied to her parents about where the money had gone—"toiletries and cosmetics"—and they believed her.

In January 2014 she stole her father's credit cards and charged $25,000 to an online site on home décor items for her apartment. She also got a speeding ticket. Both of these behaviors she now attributes to compulsive Adderall use, but her parents interpreted her behavior as a money-management issue, and they insisted she get professional help for that problem. Neither imagined that behind the stealing, speeding, and spending was an Adderall addiction.

The therapist she went to see for help with her personal finance habits discovered the Adderall addiction by using the prescription drug–monitoring database and uncovering multiple identical prescriptions from multiple doctors. This was not the first time one of her doctors had discovered her secret. When it had happened once before, the psychiatrist had refused to treat her, and so Karen moved on to another one. This time, the psychiatrist asked Karen's permission to inform her parents. Karen reluctantly agreed.

Enduring Pain Instead of Medicating It Away

Karen came to see me as the result of an ultimatum from her parents and her psychiatrist: get an evaluation by an addiction medicine doctor, or else. At first Karen wanted to talk only about her attention deficit disorder and to explain away her Adderall use as a necessary accommodation of her illness. I said, as I usually do in this kind of situation, that whatever compelled her to first start using the drug, even if it was a legitimate medical indication, had now escalated to the level of an addiction, and if we didn't target and treat the addiction, her underlying disorder would not improve either.[76] We slowly tapered her down and off of Adderall, and she attended a day-treatment program for addiction, consisting of groups, psychoeducation, and skills training related to the treatment of addiction.

Karen has been abstinent from stimulants for almost a year. Stopping Adderall hasn't been easy for her. The biggest challenge has been rewriting her personal narrative. She has had to learn to live in the world without medicating away her limitations. She has had to tolerate normal ebbs and flows of energy, subjective well-being, and creativity. She has had to accept that sometimes when she is feeling down or tired, bored or angry, sad or inattentive, she can't willfully erase those feelings. She just has to endure them.

4

Big Pharma Joins Big Medicine

Co-opting Medical Science to Promote Pill-Taking

Jim lay flat on his back in a hospital bed, morphine seeping into his veins through a long, thin, transparent tube. He felt no pain of any kind, and yet he continued to be obsessively preoccupied with his next dose of pain medication. As the time approached, he counted the minutes and seconds until he could ring the nurse and ask for more. She wouldn't just give it for free, however; he had to answer her questions the right way. She would always ask the same question before she could administer the meds: "On a scale from 1 to 10, how bad is your pain, with 0 being no pain, and 10 being the worst pain you could possibly imagine."

After years of manipulating people to manage, or attempt to manage, his drinking, Jim had developed a deep understanding of certain aspects of human psychology, especially how to appear trustworthy while lying. In this instance, he applied those skills, because he was not in fact having much if any pain by day three into his hospitalization. But he wanted those opioids.

He figured that if he said "10," he would be seen as someone who exaggerated. If he said anything less than "7," he might not get his morphine, which he already thought of as his. So he said, "My pain is real bad, it's a 7," going for the middle of the road approach as a way to appear reasonable but still sufficiently distressed. Whether due to Jim's skillful psychological manipulation or not, "7" worked every time, and Jim managed to get intravenous morphine every four hours continuously for his entire hospital stay, which lasted about a week.

There was only one moment when Jim suspected that he was in trouble. It was a conversation with one of his nurses.

"Jim," said the nurse, "You're taking a lot of this stuff, and I'm worried. I've seen so many people come through here and end up sicker than when they started because of these pain meds. They get hooked. I don't want that to happen to you. So if you could cut back, that would be good. But if you tell me you're in pain," she added, as if catching herself, "I'll give it to you every time."

Very quiet and distant alarm bells rang in Jim's brain, but they were too quiet and too distant to compete with his overwhelming craving for the next dose of morphine.

"I can handle it," he told her, "and I'm in pain."

This interaction between Jim and his nurse is crucial to understanding the rapid rise in prescription opioid addiction and opioid-related deaths. Jim's nurse knew on some level that Jim was getting too many opioids, and she even admitted to seeing patients "end up sicker than when they started" because of the amount of opioids they received while hospitalized. But despite her misgivings, she felt pressure to follow the standardized protocol: no cumulative dose or duration of opioids is too high for a patient still endorsing pain.

Curing Doctors of Their "Opioiphobia"

The prolific opioid prescribing that characterized the 1990s and 2000s and that continues today, at a galloping although somewhat slower pace, represents a radical shift in practice. Prior to 1980, doctors used opioid pain relievers sparingly, and only for the short term in cases of severe injury or illness, or during surgery.[77, 78] Their reluctance to use opioids for an extended length of time, despite their short-term effectiveness for pain, sprang from fear of causing addiction.*

In the early 1980s, however, professional medical opinion on the use of opioid pain relievers began to change, in favor of using opioids more liberally. The number of patients living with pain was growing, due to an aging population, to more people undergoing and surviving complicated surgeries, and to more people being kept alive with life-threatening illnesses. A new movement, known as hospice care, was beginning to make inroads in the United States at this time as well, advocating for more aggressive comfort care at the end of life.

What began as a good faith effort to improve the lives of patients in pain soon gave way to an epidemic of opioid painkiller overprescribing. The pharmaceutical industry (Big Pharma), specifically the makers of opioid painkillers like OxyContin (Purdue Pharma), played a pivotal role in the epidemic. But to ascribe all the blame to Big Pharma is to oversimplify. The pharmaceutical industry was able to influence doctor-prescribing only by joining together with academic physicians, professional medical societies, regulatory agencies (the Federation of State Medical Boards and The Joint Commission), and the Food and Drug Administration. Together, these different factions manipulated and misrepresented, deliberately or otherwise, medical science to serve their own agendas.

The Role of Academic Physicians

It had been common practice before 2000 for doctors to accept gifts, meals, payments, travel, and other services from companies that made

* The United States endured two opioid epidemics in the twentieth century, the first in the early 1900s, when heroin was marketed alongside Bayer aspirin as a remedy for numerous minor ailments. The second, in the 1960s, coincided with the Vietnam War and again involved mostly heroin, although by then heroin was illegal. These prior experiences with opioids made the medical community understandably reluctant to repeat history's mistakes.

the drugs and medical products they might recommend to their patients.*[79] Many of these overt attempts to influence doctors have since been banned by hospitals and other health care institutions across the country, in recognition that even a free pen and half an hour of a drug representative's time can unduly influence prescribing practices. An analysis published by the *Journal of the American Medical Association* found that doctors who accept perks from drugmakers are more likely to prescribe that drugmaker's brand of drugs.[80] Recent federal legislation demands that doctors who receive financial reimbursement from a drug or medical supply company disclose those payments. In September 2014, the Sunshine Act required that all corporate payments to physicians worth $10 or more be published in an online database, in hopes that more transparency would alert patients to which doctors might be unduly influenced by industry.[79] These changes discouraged many doctors from openly taking gifts from Big Pharma.

Big Pharma responded by changing tactics. Instead of influencing doctor-prescribing by giving perks directly to doctors, it instead enlisted the help of academic researchers to promote its products, while itself remaining invisible, in the background. Big Pharma dubbed these doctors "thought leaders," choosing only researchers whose results favored their drug. They paid for thought leaders to travel across the country presenting their work at medical conferences and so-called informational seminars. Pharmaceutical companies were careful not to overtly associate their thought leader's message with their brand. They often paid thought leaders large sums of money to speak, and in some

---

*The pharmaceutical industry also engages in direct-to-consumer advertising, that is, it markets to patient consumers directly. Most people are familiar with Pharma ads on TV promoting better sleep, hotter sex (or for the middle-aged and older, any sex at all), less pain, and more joy. These commercials frequently depict an ecstatic woman running through a field of springtime flowers, butterflies alighting on her shoulders, and ending with the phrase "Ask your doctor if drug X is right for you." This kind of advertising can influence prescribing because doctors are eager to please their patients, and when a patient asks about a particular medication, a doctor may prescribe it over other comparable choices.

instances provided the funds to subsidize the entire medical conference/seminar. They promoted the drug company's product, while also furthering their elected thought leader's academic career.

This insidious yet incredibly powerful method—what amounts to a Trojan Horse of drug peddling—represents a betrayal of the average doctor seeing patients. The average clinician relies on his or her academic colleagues to present unbiased research. When the average doctor attends an academic conference, he or she trusts that the organizers of the conference will feature speakers who represent diverse and scientifically valid viewpoints.

New York Times journalist Barry Meier, in his excellent book *Pain Killer*,[81] describes how Big Pharma chose Dr. Russell Portenoy as their "thought leader," supporting his travel around the country to promote more liberal opioid prescribing for many types of pain. Dr. Portenoy's talks were sponsored by drug companies or by the Dannemiller Foundation, an organization paid by drug companies to put on continuing medical education programs for doctors. Dr. Portenoy had financial relationships with at least a dozen companies, most of which produced prescription opioids.[81]

The first misconception about opioid painkillers conveyed to doctors by Dr. Portenoy and others is that these drugs are effective for the treatment of chronic pain (pain lasting three or more months). The benefit of short-term opioid therapy is supported by multiple clinical trials,[82] but there is very little evidence to support the use of opioids for managing chronic pain, and the risks of long-term use may outweigh the benefits.[83] One of the risks, paradoxically, may be an increase in pain due to a phenomenon called "opioid induced hyperalgesia" (OIH), "hyper" for "more/over," and "algesia" for "pain." Animal and human studies show that prolonged use of opioid painkillers can cause heightened sensitivity to pain and result in pain syndromes that did not previously exist.[84] One small prospective study of six patients with chronic lower back pain started on oral morphine demonstrated that all six developed hyperalgesia (increased sensitivity to pain) after four weeks.[85]

The second misconception is that no dose of opioid painkillers is too high for the treatment of pain. In fact, we know that tolerance to the pain-relieving effects of opioids occurs in most individuals after weeks to months, at which point the opioids stop working, no matter how high the dose. The risk of side effects, however, rises in a dose-depending manner[83]—the higher the dose, the worse the side effects, including the risks of addiction and death due to accidental overdose.

Dr. Portenoy based his false assertions on a study he had published in 1986 with Dr. Kathleen Foley in a medical journal simply called *Pain*. The study was a review of thirty-eight patients with chronic pain treated with opioid painkillers. Portenoy and Foley wrote that "opioid maintenance therapy can be a safe, salutary and more humane alternative . . . in those patients with intractable non-malignant pain and no history of drug abuse."[86] This statement represents a plea for a departure from previous practice, in which opioids were used almost exclusively for acute (after surgery or injury) and palliative (at the end of life) pain. The authors also go on to say that no amount of opioids to treat chronic pain is too much, again flying in the face of convention, which had always advocated using the bare minimum to avoid the risks of death due to respiratory suppression and addiction: "We disagree with the concept of setting a maximum dose. The pharmacology of opioid use in the treatment of pain is based on dose titration to effect."[86]

Portenoy and Foley's review of thirty-eight patients does not, however, constitute a high level of scientific evidence. It did not include a large number of patients. There was no comparison group taking a placebo or getting some other treatment for pain, such as physical therapy. It was retrospective rather than prospective, meaning that the authors asked patients to recollect past experiences, biased by recall effects, rather than soliciting their reactions going forward in real time. Although these patients endorsed improvements in pain with opioids, they did not report any functional improvement. Yet this study became very well known in the medical community, and its publication and dissemination correlated with a sudden uptick in the rate of opioid prescriptions for patients with chronic pain.[87]

As Portenoy's talks drew ever larger crowds, he frequently referenced other publications that supported his view.[81] He invoked a 1980 *New England Journal of Medicine* letter to the editor entitled "Addiction Rare in Patients Treated with Narcotics." The letter reported that among hospitalized patients taking opioids for pain, clinical researchers had found "only four cases of addiction among 11,882 patients treated with opioids."[46] This letter was widely cited by doctors and medical organizations and frequently quoted by the pharmaceutical industry in its advertisements for opioids, as proving that "less-than-1%" of patients receiving opioids for pain become addicted.[81] This misconception—that as long as doctors were prescribing opioids for the treatment of pain, there was less than a 1 percent chance of their patients becoming addicted—was perhaps the most egregious. It implied that the well-known inherent addictive potential of opioids was magically eliminated by the halo of a doctor's prescription. We know now that opioid painkillers prescribed by a doctor are as addictive as heroin purchased on a street corner.

The final misconception perpetuated by the pseudoscience of this era was the idea of "pseudoaddiction." Based on a single case report of a patient who engaged in drug-seeking behavior due to inadequate pain control,[88] doctors were taught that any patient prescribed opioid painkillers who demonstrates drug seeking behavior is not addicted, but in pain. The solution? Increase the dose of opioid painkillers. We know that many patients have severe debilitating pain, and sometimes the appropriate intervention is to increase the opioid painkillers. But some patients who report pain and are engaging in drug-seeking behavior are addicted to opioids. They may also have untreated pain. To help this population, doctors need to recognize and treat both disorders, not ignore the possibility of addiction.

In a taped interview with Dr. Russell Portenoy in 2011, on the website for the advocacy group Physicians for Responsible Opioid Prescribing (PROP),[89] Portenoy describes his unabashed advocacy for opioids in the 1990s and early 2000s as follows: "I gave so many lectures to primary care audiences in which the Porter and Jick article[46] was just one piece of data that I would then cite. I would cite 6 to 7 maybe 10 different avenues of thought or evidence, none of which represents real evidence. And yet what I was trying to do was to create a narrative so that the primary care audience would look at this information in toto and feel more comfortable about opioids in a way they hadn't before. . . . Because the primary goal was to de-stigmatize, we often left evidence behind."[89]

The Role of Professional Medical Societies

Every medical specialty, from family medicine to orthopedic surgery, has medical societies created by and for the doctors who practice it. The purpose of a medical society is to promote the specialty and its doctors and also, theoretically, to advocate for patients.

Beginning in the 1980s, pain societies campaigned for better treatment of patients with pain, including arguing for more liberal use of opioid painkillers in the treatment of pain. On the face of it, their intentions were noble. But closer scrutiny reveals that some of these pain societies were financially subsidized by drug manufacturers and as such were biased. They helped propagate data that turned out to be untrue, including minimizing the risk of addiction to opioid painkillers prescribed for pain and inflating the number of Americans struggling with pain. They also influenced the creation of a new stigmatized identity: the doctor unwilling to prescribe opioids for patients in pain.

The American Pain Foundation, a medical society for doctors who treat pain, received 90 percent of its $5 million funding in 2010 from the drug and medical device industry. The extent to which other pain societies might have been subsidized by Big Pharma is unclear, but according to an article published in *ProPublica* in 2012, US senators Baucus and Grassley launched an investigation into the American Pain Foundation, the American Academy of Pain Medicine, the American Pain Society, the Wisconsin Pain and Policy Group, and the Center for Practical Bioethics, exploring the extent to which drug manufacturers such as Purdue Pharma, Endo Pharmaceuticals, and Johnson and Johnson might have encouraged these societies to promote opioid painkiller prescribing.[90]

The American Pain Society, founded in 1995 with Dr. Portenoy as its first president, issued treatment guidelines urging doctors to prescribe more opioids for the treatment of pain. Their self-proclaimed goal was to cure the medical community of its "opioiphobia" (fear of prescribing opioids). The American Pain Society and the American Academy of Pain Medicine published a consensus statement in 1997 which proclaimed there was insufficient evidence to conclude that opioids, when prescribed for the treatment of pain, can result in opioid addiction.[91]

In 2011, the Institute of Medicine (IOM) committee, commissioned by the US Congress, issued a report called "Relieving Pain in America." In it, they declared that 100 million Americans—nearly a third of the population—suffer from chronic debilitating pain, at a cost of $600 billion a year in medical treatments and lost productivity.[92] They also claimed that a "cultural transformation" was necessary to improve pain management. However, the number 100 million was an exaggeration, the real number being closer to 25 million Americans with debilitating pain, or approximately 15 percent of the population.[93] Twenty-five million is still a high number of individuals in pain, and these patients need and deserve medical attention. But the cultural transformation the IOM report demanded had already occurred, to the point that doctors were engaging in excessive opioid prescribing.

In 2010 the International Association for the Study of Pain (IASP) issued a declaration stating that all patients are entitled to "access to pain management without discrimination . . . on the basis of age, sex, gender, medical diagnosis, race or ethnicity, religion, culture, marital, civil, or socioeconomic status, sexual orientation, and political or other opinions"; and "appropriate treatment includes access to pain medications, including opioids and other essential medications for pain."[94] This statement reads more like a patient bill of rights than a policy guideline, illustrating how the campaign to destigmatize the use of opioid therapy turned into a campaign to stigmatize any doctor who wasn't prescribing opioids for pain. Opioids, doctors were told, needed to be prescribed for all forms of pain, at ever-increasing doses, lest the doctors risk engaging in unethical, discriminatory practices.

The Role of the Federation of State Medical Boards

The Federation of State Medical Boards (FSMB) is a national organization that oversees the seventy medical and osteopathic boards of the United States and its territories. The state board organizations serve many functions, one of which is to police doctors and exert disciplinary action against doctors who are deemed dangerous to patients. One of the most severe forms of disciplinary action is to revoke a doctor's license to practice medicine.

In 1998, the FSMB issued a policy to reassure doctors that they would not be prosecuted if they prescribed even large amounts of opioids, as long as it was for the treatment of pain. In 2001, every licensed physician in the state of California was mandated to attend a day-long course on the treatment of pain as a requirement to maintain licensure. The federation urged state medical boards to punish doctors for undertreating pain. Doctors lived in fear of disciplinary action from the board, and the lawsuit that usually followed, if they denied a patient opioid painkillers. In 1991 in North Carolina, in the case of *Henry James v. Hillhaven*, $7.5 million was granted to the family because a nurse did not follow the doctor's order to properly address pain. In 1998 in California in the case of *Bergman v. Eden Medical Center*, $1.5 million was granted to the family because the physician did not properly address the patient's pain.

The FSMB published a book promoting the use of opioid painkillers. This book was funded by Purdue Pharma, Endo Health Solutions, and others, with proceeds totaling $280,000, and was developed with the help of David Haddox, a senior Purdue Pharma executive.[81] The federation admitted to receiving nearly $2 million dollars from opioid makers since 1997 to support its efforts.[81]

The Role of the Joint Commission on Accreditation of Healthcare Organizations

The Joint Commission on Accreditation of Healthcare Organizations (JCAHO), often simply referred to as "The Joint Commission" (TJC), is a United States–based nonprofit tax-exempt 501(c) organization that accredits health care organizations and programs in the United States. The Joint Commission arose out of a movement in the 1950s to reform hospitals by looking at whether or not patients got better. JCAHO went through a consolidation of power over the years, combining multiple medical organizations under one roof, simplifying its name in 2007 to "The Joint Commission." Its mission statement is "Helping Health Care Organizations Help Patients."

Today, having Joint Commission accreditation is required for many hospitals and clinics to remain licensed. Payment for services from the Centers for Medicare and Medicaid Services (CMS), the largest federally funded insurance program, is also contingent on TJC approval. TJC approval is obtained through periodic surveys. Huge amounts of time and large sums of money are devoted to preparing for these surveys, which hospitals must pay TJC to perform.

These surveys assess adherence to "best practices." Best practices are defined by TJC itself: "Joint Commission standards are developed with input from health care professionals, providers, subject matter experts, consumers, government agencies (including the Centers for Medicare & Medicaid Services) and employers. They are informed by scientific literature and expert consensus and reviewed by the Board of Commissioners. New standards are added only if they relate to patient safety or quality of care, have a positive impact on health outcomes, meet or surpass law and regulation, and can be accurately and readily measured."[95]

In 2001, The Joint Commission made "pain" the fifth vital sign, alongside heart rate, temperature, respiratory rate, and blood pressure, indicating the state of a patient's essential body functions. Pain, however, unlike the original vital signs, cannot be objectively measured. Thus, TJC promoted the use of the Visual Analog Scale of pain assessment (a series of happy and sad faces corresponding to degrees of pain), accompanied by a number on a scale from 1 to 10, with 10 out of 10 pain being the worst pain a human being could endure and 1 the pain equivalent of, let's say, a stubbed toe. Quantifying pain made it possible to standardize procedures across doctors and met TJC's own requirement of implementing new standards only if they could "be accurately and readily measured."

Despite the appearance of objectivity, the Visual Analog Scale and the numerical pain scale represent entirely arbitrary measurements. There is in fact no way to measure a person's pain. One person's severed leg might be a 1 on the pain scale, and another person's stubbed toe a 10. Furthermore, no scientific studies show that using these pain scales correlates with improved patient outcomes. Data do show, however, that use of these pain scores increases opioid prescribing and opioid use.[96, 97]

The Joint Commission launched a nationwide "pain management educational program." They sold educational materials to hospitals so they could meet the standards of pain treatment that would be required to pass the next Joint Commission Survey.[98] These materials included laminated cards and posters of the Visual Analog Scale of pain, as well as teaching videos promoting more liberal prescribing of opioids for pain: "Some clinicians have inaccurate and exaggerated concerns about addiction, tolerance and risk of death. . . . This attitude prevails despite the fact there is no evidence that addiction is a significant issue when persons are given opioids for pain control."[99] Many of these teaching materials were produced by Purdue Pharma, the makers of OxyContin, and given to TJC, free of charge.

A Government Accountability Report, published in 2003, had this to say about the relationship between TJC (herein referred to as JCAHO) and Purdue Pharma:

> From 1996, when OxyContin was introduced to the market, to July 2002, Purdue has funded over 20,000 pain-related educational programs through direct sponsorship or financial grants. These grants included support for programs to provide physicians with opportunities to earn required continuing medical education credits, such as grand round presentations at hospitals and medical education seminars at state and local medical conferences. During 2001 and 2002, Purdue funded a series of nine programs throughout the country to educate hospital physicians and staff on how to comply with JCAHO's pain standards for hospitals and to discuss postoperative pain treatment. Purdue was one of only two drug companies that provided funding for JCAHO's pain management educational programs. Under an agreement with JCAHO, Purdue was the only drug company allowed to distribute certain educational videos and a book about pain management; these materials were also available for purchase from JCAHO's Web site. Purdue's participation in these activities with JCAHO may have facilitated its access to hospitals to promote OxyContin. [98]

In 2012, The Joint Commission published a report on the safe use of opioids in hospitals, publicly recognizing the need for improved patient assessment and management to lower the incidence of opioid overdose in the inpatient setting.[100]

The Role of the Food and Drug Administration

The Food and Drug Administration (FDA) is an agency within the US Department of Health and Human Services responsible for assuring the safety, effectiveness, and quality of medical drugs. They are responsible for approving drugs before they reach the market and monitoring the safety and marketing of those drugs once they have become available to the public. The FDA contributed to the prescription opioid painkiller epidemic by failing to prevent drug companies from promoting opioid painkillers in the treatment of chronic pain, for which there was little evidence, and by making it easier for pharmaceutical companies to get FDA approval for new opioids coming on the market.

Every pharmaceutical company that seeks FDA approval for a particular drug must demonstrate to the FDA in a series of clinical trials (studies) that their drug is better than a placebo (a sugar pill) and that, whatever side effects posed by the drug, the potential benefits (for a given population of patients) outweigh the risks. In the late 1990s, the FDA implemented a new study protocol for FDA approval called "enriched enrollment," which it said would result in smaller studies, shortened drug development time, and lower development costs for the pharmaceutical industry. The investigative journalist John Fauber, writing for the *Wisconsin Sentinel*, said the decision to change study requirements arose from a series of meetings over more than a decade between experts in pain medicine, primarily from academia, and representatives of the FDA. The invitation-only meetings were sponsored by Big Pharma, which paid up to $35,000 for drug company representatives to attend, raising "serious questions about the way in which federal regulators interact with the pharmaceutical companies they regulate."[101] The enriched enrollment protocol does appear to be a way for drug companies to cheat, getting approval for opioid painkillers that don't really work.

In traditional studies that assess the benefit of a drug as compared with a placebo, participants are randomly assigned to participate in one group or the other. The random assignment of the participants is fundamental to good clinical studies because it insures that neither group is predisposed to do better, or worse, on the drug or placebo, than the other. With this traditional design, opioid medications in the treatment of chronic pain were not performing well. This was happening for a number of reasons. First, a lot of patients on opioids were dropping out of the study due to side effects, such as dizziness, constipation, nausea, or vomiting. Second, participants in the placebo group were doing better, in part because they weren't having the side effects. Placebo, it turns out, is pretty good medication for chronic pain. Drug companies were understandably frustrated because they were not getting the results necessary for FDA approval. So the study design was revised. The new design, which persists today, is called "enriched enrollment."

With enriched enrollment, instead of giving half of the participants the study drug and half the placebo, investigators give everyone the study drug in what is called the "open-label phase," because both researchers and participants can see the metaphorical label on the pill bottle and know the subject is getting an opioid. During this open-label phase, as many as half of the participants typically drop out due to side effects and opioid intolerance, or maybe just because opioids are not a good medicine for chronic pain. The people left in the study are all the people who are on some level benefitting from the opioids. At the end of the open-label phase, all the participants are tapered down and off opioids, and re-randomized to two groups, opioid or placebo.

Enriched enrollment is a flawed design because the study population is not generalizable to all chronic pain patients but only to chronic pain patients who already like opioids. The study is also no longer double blind because the participants who continue to experience opioid withdrawal, which can go on for weeks and months in some people, continue to feel worse when they're randomized to placebo. What naturally ends up happening is that many of the individuals who liked being on opioids and who are randomized to placebo end up dropping out of the study, so now the dropout rate is higher in the placebo arm than in the study-drug arm. The result is that the opioid study drug ends up looking better than placebo, and the drug gets approved by the FDA.

Here's an analogy. Imagine you are testing a theory that, to keep kids happy and well-behaved during lunchtime recess, playing soccer is better than engaging in arts and crafts. You take the entire third-grade class and randomly, by drawing names from a hat, divide the students into two groups: half to play soccer and half to sit at the arts and crafts table and make hand puppets. At the end, you use some measure to assess whether kids are happier and better behaved when they play soccer or when they do art. That is a classic randomized study design.

Now suppose that instead of the above, you make all the kids play soccer every day at lunch for two weeks first, before randomizing them to different groups. Naturally, the kids who already like soccer or are more athletic or have higher energy will probably enjoy this. The kids who are naturally unathletic, low-energy, or disinclined to play sports will not like this. In fact, quite a few of them may simply refuse to participate and may even bring in notes from their parents asking that they be allowed to sit out during lunch. At the end of the two weeks, you might have only half the number of kids still playing soccer because the rest have dropped out of the study. All clinical studies have subjects who drop out, ending with many fewer subjects than when the study started.

With the kids left, most of whom enjoy soccer, you now randomly assign half to soccer, and half to arts and crafts. The kids who get randomized to soccer are happy. The ones who get randomized to arts and crafts are not so happy. They miss soccer and are now also fidgety and restless because their bodies had gotten used to getting exercise during lunch. Your study results unequivocally show that kids who play soccer are much happier and better behaved than kids who do arts and crafts, and every school in the district, as a result of your work, has mandatory soccer at lunchtime.

The FDA has made some limited innovations to target the prescription opioid epidemic, but for every step forward, they've taken two back. In 2014, the FDA reclassified Vicodin, among the most misused painkillers in the 1990s and early 2000s, to schedule II, making it harder for doctors to prescribe it and hence for patients to get it.[102] But nearly simultaneously, in 2013, the FDA approved Zohydro, a long-acting version of Vicodin that is likely to be as addictive as or more addictive than

Vicodin. The FDA is meanwhile keeping drugs like Opana on the market. Opana was approved in 2011 as an "abuse-deterrent" opioid painkiller, but since then has proven to be highly addictive when injected. It was recently tied to a 2015 outbreak of HIV in rural Indiana, as well as a surge in hepatitis C infections in Kentucky, Tennessee, West Virginia, and Virginia.

The Engine and the Caboose

In 2007 three of Purdue's top executives pleaded guilty to "misbranding" OxyContin as less addictive than it is, and Purdue paid $634 million in fines, the eleventh largest fine paid by a pharmaceutical firm in the history of the US Department of Justice. Of the fines paid by Purdue in 2007, about $160 million went to reimburse the federal government and some states for damages suffered by Medicaid programs, the government health insurer for the poor.[103]

Kentucky, one of the states especially hard hit by the prescription opioid epidemic, refused its reimbursement of $500,000, the only state to do so, deciding instead to file its own class action lawsuit against Purdue. Similar class action suits have been filed by Illinois and California. When Kentucky's suit against Purdue goes to trial, it will be an unprecedented event. Purdue Pharma has never gone to trial for OxyContin and has succeeded in dismissing more than four hundred personal injury lawsuits related to the use of OxyContin. If Kentucky wins, Purdue is facing an extraordinary fine, comparable to the class action suits that cost Big Tobacco billions in the 1990s. Unfortunately, it's too little too late for the 175,000 people who have died from prescription opioid overdose between 1999 and 2013, not to mention the lives lost before and after.

Manufacturers of opioid painkillers have contributed to the opioid epidemic that has ravaged the United States, but blame cannot be placed on Big Pharma alone. Blame lies with doctors as well, especially those in academia and other positions of leadership who ignored the evidence on risk and efficacy in pursuit of their own agenda—an agenda that originated in a desire to help but then lost its way. Blame also lies with regulatory agencies like the Federation of State Medical Boards, The Joint Commission, and the FDA, which blindly followed the lead of the pharmaceutical industry, propagated misinformation, and failed to do their jobs: to regulate.

Big Medicine was the engine behind the opioid paradigm shift, and Big Pharma the stealthy and powerful caboose. Big Medicine provided legitimacy, and Big Pharma the funds to push the message along. Neither anticipated the success of their partnership, nor the runaway train it would become when the opioid epidemic took over.

5

The Drug-Seeking Patient

Malingering versus the Hijacked Brain

Jim was discharged from the hospital with a peripherally inserted central catheter, or PICC line, in place to allow for prolonged intravenous access for the antibiotics he would continue to take in subsequent months to treat his infection. Weeks later, Jim would discover that the PICC line was useful for other reasons as well.

He was given a prescription for a one-month supply of Norco, a combination of acetaminophen (Tylenol) and the highly addictive opioid hydrocodone (the primary ingredient in Vicodin). Within one week Jim was taking more Norco than prescribed, and he was prescribed two pills every four hours, a considerable dose to begin with. Within three weeks, his month's supply was gone, and he was back at the same hospital emergency room asking for more.

Six months after his hospitalization, Jim was ingesting 600 morphine mg equivalents* of opioids per day. Enough to kill a baby ele-

---

*Conversions and comparisons between different opioids is typically accomplished by estimating the equivalent dose of oral morphine, often referred to as morphine milligram equivalents, or MME. For example, 10 mg of oral oxycodone is approximately equal to 15 mg of oral morphine, or 15 MME.

phant? A person who had never taken an opioid or anyone who had not taken opioids for an extended length of time would likely die taking the dose Jim was taking daily, but Jim's body and brain had built up such tolerance to the effect of opioids that, at this point, he needed to take that much every day just to stave off withdrawal. If he ran out, he experienced opioid withdrawal, including nausea, diarrhea, insomnia, irritability, anxiety, and painful muscle cramps—the last being the origin of the phrase "kicking the habit."

He told himself he was taking the medication to treat his low back pain, and therefore he "deserved it." He told himself he'd quit tomorrow, that he had it under control, and that it wouldn't be like alcohol. Meanwhile, he could think of nothing except obtaining and using pain pills.

By 2013, Jim was spending hours a day going around to different doctors' offices, sometimes multiple doctors in one day, but never the same one within two weeks, looking for prescriptions for Norco and other similar medications—oxycodone, OxyContin, Vicodin, Percocet, all containing the same essential active ingredient: opioids. The phenomenon of patients like Jim going around to multiple health care providers to obtain prescription drugs is referred to as "doctor shopping." The trick, Jim found, was to find clinics that advertised "walk-ins" and "no appointment necessary" because they were accustomed to patients they'd never met before showing up for treatment.

Jim's unassuming appearance worked to his advantage. He typically wore a T-shirt and track pants, always very clean, and white socks with white sneakers. His short, dyed black hair gave him a slight resemblance to Ronald Reagan. He was not too tall or too short, too fat or too thin, too rich or too poor. He was average, likable, and forgettable.

He exaggerated his symptoms and attempted to validate his medical claim with objective medical evidence. He got a cane and mastered a convincing limp. He armed himself with a paper copy of his official discharge summary, documenting his medical workup, and he made sure to wear a short-sleeve shirt so his PICC line was clearly visible. He'd tell his doctors he was still on IV antibiotics, though the need for the antibiotics had long since passed, and the PICC line was by now a prop rather than a needed medical device. At each visit, he described his prior treatments and mentioned the doctors who had treated him in the past by name because, he sensed, using a specific name legitimized his story. If the doctors recognized the names, that was even better.

He sought above all to be likable and sympathetic. He seldom mentioned any drug specifically, deferring to the doctors to come up with it themselves. He talked about the terrible pain he was in, gesturing, with a wince in the direction of his low back and legs.

He knew the doctors would have questions, and he was ready for them:

"Why aren't you seeing your primary care doctor about this problem?"

"He retired." "She's on maternity leave." "He won't treat pain."

"What else have you tried for your pain?"

"Tylenol, ibuprofen, aspirin, acupuncture, trigger-point injections, physical therapy—nothing works."

"What are your long-term goals in terms of pain management?"

"I don't want to take medications. I want to get off this stuff. I want to get better. But the pain is just so terrible right now . . . "

Jim used several different strategies to get the drugs he wanted. He was charming, conciliatory, never pushy, and he lied. He exaggerated his symptoms. He claimed to be getting treatment he was not getting or had never gotten. He made promises about quitting he had no intention of keeping.

Strategies Drug-Seeking Patients Use to Get Drugs

Patients use many different strategies to manipulate doctors to get the drugs they want. The myriad ways drug-seeking patients effectively manipulate doctors can be codified into distinct categories, or personas. These labels are not intended to denigrate drug-seeking patients but to capture complex behavior in memorable ways.

Sycophants. Sycophants are patients who flatter and cajole, assuring their doctor of their competence and compassion, especially as compared to that of every other doctor they've seen. The patient satisfaction surveys give this technique additional leverage because the communication goes beyond just the doctor and the patient. It is unveiled for the larger institution to see, and sometimes the whole Internet world, as in the case of Web-based doctor-rating platforms that use patient ratings as the only measure.

Senators. Senators are patients who use the filibuster technique, taking most of the allotted time with the doctor to talk about issues unrelated to the prescription, intentionally waiting until the last few minutes of the encounter to bring it up. In doing so, they are relying on the time pressures they know the doctor is under to tip the doctor over into prescribing because it is the expedient thing to do. Saying yes to a prescription and ordering it takes less than one minute. Saying no could take thirty minutes or more, much less time than the doctor has to stay on schedule.

Exhibitionists. Exhibitionists are patients who display intense emotions and dramatic gestures associated with refill requests. Sometimes they writhe in pain. Other times they achieve various stages of undress to reveal colostomy bags, surgical scars, congenital deformities. The heightened theatrics are intended to illustrate a sense of dire need. As one patient said to me regarding my ability to prescribe him the drugs he was requesting, "I'm on fire, and you've got the hose."

Losers. Losers are patients who exhibit a remarkable tendency to misplace medications. With astonishing regularity, these patients run their medication in the wash cycle, drop them over the side of the fishing boat, flush them down the toilet—water seems to be a common theme. There's also leaving them in a hotel room, being parted from them as a result of lost luggage during a weekend getaway, and yes, I have even heard of meds being eaten by the family pet.

Weekenders. Weekenders call for early refills or increased dosages when their regular doctors, the ones who know them best, are least likely to be around. Academic medical centers, where less-experienced trainees are most likely to get calls off-hours, are particularly vulnerable to this technique. Large health care conglomerates where shift work is the norm also fall prey.

Doctor Shoppers. Doctor shoppers are patients who go to multiple doctors simultaneously for the same or similar prescriptions. These patients seek out clinics where drop-in visits are welcome, and where doctors are accustomed to seeing a patient once and possibly never again. Emergency rooms provide the ultimate one-stop shopping, because they are staffed by many different doctors. According to one study, doctor shoppers seeking prescription opioids are more likely to be between 26 and 35 years of age, to pay for prescriptions with cash, and to obtain oxycodone formulations (2.8 percent), followed by oxymorphone (2.3 percent), followed by tramadol (2.0 percent).[104]

Impersonators. Impersonators are patients who assume different identities at different clinics or hospitals—the inverse of doctor shopping. Instead of searching around for different doctors, they become different people.

Dynamic Duo. The Dynamic Duos are patients who present in teams of two, usually the patient and the patient's mother, the commonest codependent. While the patient is writhing in pain, the patient's mother is crying. Together they make a formidable and persuasive team.

Twins. Twins are the patients who are also health care providers or who occupy a professional and social class that the doctor relates to. These patients know how to create a sense of affiliation with the doctor by talking about the schools they went to, the high-level jobs they've had or have, the people they may know in common. The ones who are health care providers use their intimate knowledge of the health care system to encourage their doctors to prescribe for them.

Country Mice and City Mice. Country mice and city mice are patients who situate themselves on the opposite ends of the savvy spectrum. The country mouse is the faux naïf, and the city mouse the slicker. The country mouse pretends to know nothing about prescription medication and gently persuades the doctor to suggest the drugs. The city mouse, by contrast, saunters into the emergency room and announces she is allergic to all pain medications except intravenous Dilaudid push (the "push" meaning the syringe with the opioid medication is emptied into the bloodstream all at once to create an immediate high) with a Benadryl chaser (Benadryl is an antihistamine known to augment the high of opioids). A nurse practitioner I interviewed told me that she once treated a city mouse who was so resistant to transitioning from the intravenous Dilaudid push, given to him in the emergency room, to the oral or rectal opioid she offered him once he had been admitted to the floor, that he left the hospital without further treatment.

Bullies. Bullies are patients who use emotional or even physical intimidation to coerce doctors to prescribe. Bullying may represent one of the most effective techniques. These patients have a deep understanding of the fears that plague doctors—the fear of a negative review, the fear of litigation. Patients exploit these fears to serve their own agendas.

Internet Copycats. Internet copycats use the Internet to obtain information on how to get drugs from doctors. A Google query of "How to trick dr's to give u pain medicine" gives the following result. "The trick—seriously—is to visit a poor doctor in a poor area of town. Get your textbook list of requirements, pay cash for your appointment, and be the perfect patient. Each time, ask for a little bit more painkillers for a little bit more pain. The doctors want to cover their asses legally and not go to jail or get sued, but it's no hair off their back if you're a lifetime pain mgmt candidate." And "Just look up bullsh——t medical problems like fibromyalgia symptoms and go to the doctor and tell him/her that is how you feel. Fibromyalgia is just a made up medical term for people that want pain killers."

Little Engines That Could. Little engines are patients who plod along, always communicating enough improvement to convince the doctor they're almost there, almost over the hump, while endorsing enough ongoing distress to continue to receive the desired prescription. These are the same patients who say "I really want to get off these meds" but never take the necessary steps to make that happen.

Understanding the Drug-Seeking Patient

For the purposes of this discussion, the drug-seeking patient is the patient who attempts to obtain a medication from a doctor for his or her own nontherapeutic or addictive use, not the drug-seeking patient who plans to give or sell the medication to others (drug diversion).

The prevailing explanation for drug seeking is to accuse the patient of malingering. According to the *Diagnostic and Statistical Manual of Mental Disorders* (DSM), the reigning compendium for describing and subclassifying mental illness, malingering is "feigning illness with the conscious intent of obtaining some tangible good not related to illness recovery." Malingerers are often seeking a hot meal and shelter (referred to in medical slang as "three hots and a cot"), a disability payment, and/or prescription drugs for nontherapeutic use. Patients who are malingering represent one of the very few instances in medicine in which doctors can refuse care.

But malingering does not fully capture the phenomenon of drug seeking. Yes, drug-seeking patients lie and manipulate their doctors, and they do so knowingly. But if drugs were really all that mattered, they could obtain them with greater ease from a street dealer or an Internet pharmacy in less time and often for less money.

The drug-seeking patient is better understood through the lens of addiction. Addiction is an altered brain state in which motivation for basic survival has been "hijacked" by the drive to obtain and use substances. The invocation of the hijacked brain, a common contemporary metaphor to describe addiction, raises important philosophical questions about the role of choice, will, and moral responsibility among patients who are seeking drugs. Dr. Nora Volkow, the director of the National Institute of Drug Abuse and one of the most vocal proponents of the hijacked brain model of addiction, has likened the addicted drug-seeking patient to a starving individual looking for food. If you hadn't eaten for three days, she says, you too might do things you previously never would have considered, actions completely outside your moral compass, just to obtain a morsel of bread.

Neuroadaptation and the Pleasure-Pain Balance

To understand the neuroscience to support the idea of the hijacked brain of addiction, imagine that the brain has within it an old-fashioned scale with a straight metal beam atop a fulcrum and equally weighted platforms on each side. The job of the scale is to register and communicate pleasure and pain. When the beam is tipped down to the left, the brain senses pleasure. When the beam is tipped down to the right, the brain senses pain. When nothing is on the platforms, the beam is level with the ground and balanced, that is, homeostatic, registering neither pleasure nor pain.

According to George Koob, a neuroscientist who has spent his career studying the neuroadaptive changes the brain undergoes with chronic exposure to addictive substances, the preferred position of the beam is level, in which neither side outweighs the other. To achieve and maintain this state of equilibrium, the brain is constantly adjusting and readjusting on a biochemical level. When an individual who likes chocolate eats a piece of chocolate, the metaphorical beam tips down to the left, communicating pleasure, mediated by release of the neurotransmitter dopamine. But the scale wants to be level again. To achieve a level state, metaphorical brain gremlins start jumping on the opposite side of the scale. This might translate into decreasing the amount of pleasure-boosting dopamine the brain makes or decreasing neuronal receptors that recognize dopamine. Hence the pleasure from eating chocolate is short-lived, and the beam is level again. The brain has now "adapted" to chocolate, and the second piece doesn't taste nearly as good as the first one did.

Drugs and alcohol release much more extracellular dopamine than chocolate. When drugs and alcohol are consumed, the metaphorical beam tips much further to the left than it did with a piece of chocolate. The result is not just pleasure, but euphoria—a high. In the healthy brain, lots of brain gremlins have to pile onto the opposite side of the scale to balance it again.

Now imagine that an addictive substance is consumed for days and weeks on end. The gremlins need to work very hard to compensate, making lots of adjustments on the cellular and neurological level to keep the scale balanced. The result, over time, is a brain that is significantly altered from baseline.

What happens if the individual decides he or she no longer wants to ingest the substance or can no longer obtain it in adequate amounts to challenge the gremlins? The weight on the left side of the beam is removed, and the scale begins tipping to the right. The gremlins frantically begin dismounting, but there are so many of them that they can't go fast enough, and hence the scale passes right through equilibrium and continues tipping to the right. When the scale is tipped to the right, the individual experiences pain. This pain manifests in the form of acute physical withdrawal, but more importantly, it is associated with the emotional pain of protracted psychological withdrawal, including depression, anxiety, irritability, and insomnia, which can go on for weeks, months, and in some cases, years. This pain is so intense and overwhelming that it compels repeat drug use, not to feel high but just to equilibrate the beam and feel normal. Koob calls this "dysphoria-driven" relapse.[17]

Tincture of time (most often weeks to months) eventually allows all the gremlins to dismount the beam, at which point the beam is level, and homeostasis has been reestablished. But until that occurs, the only way some addicted persons will be able to arrive at that place is to be put in a restricted environment where they do not have access to drugs—a residential treatment center, a wilderness setting, a closed therapeutic boarding school. A commonly accepted, yet often faulty approach to dealing with addicted patients is to use the Stages of Change Model (precontemplation, contemplation, preparation, action, maintenance) and ask them if they are "ready" to take "action" to stop their addiction. If you ask an addicted patient if they are ready for treatment while their scale is still tipped to the right and their thoughts and emotions have been hijacked by the physiologic compulsion to use drugs, their answer will not reflect their true thoughts and feelings, but rather the voice of their addiction. I have seen countless patients who, in the throes of acute withdrawal, have declined addiction treatment, but who even three days later, once the acute withdrawal has passed, express an authentic desire for treatment.

Some individuals, however, may never be able to level their tipped scale and reassert homeostasis in their reward pathway. Their scales may be, in effect, broken, due to irreversible brain damage that can theoretically be caused by long-term drug use. These are the same individuals, so the rationale goes, who may benefit from long-term therapy with opioid agonist treatment (methadone or Suboxone) as a way to level the beam.

The Rationale for Methadone and Suboxone

The practice of giving an opioid to treat opioid use disorders is one that began in the United States more than fifty years ago. Two doctors, Vincent Dole and Marie Nyswander, who happened to be married to each other, published a groundbreaking study in 1967, in which they demonstrated that they could improve the lives of persons with severe heroin addiction by giving them daily doses of methadone, a synthetic opioid (made in the laboratory). Unlike heroin, which lasts for only a short time (a few hours) before the individual begins to experience painful opioid withdrawal, the effects of methadone last at least a day, thereby bridging the gap from one daily dose to the other. Thus, individuals who have developed tolerance to and dependence on opioids, and who need opioids just to feel normal, can take methadone once a day to achieve balance (homeostasis). Dole and Nyswander observed that heroin-addicted individuals whose lives had been overtaking by drug-seeking behavior could, with methadone, apply their efforts to the everyday tasks of living.

> Drug-seeking behavior, like theft, is observed after addiction is established and the narcotic drug has become euphorigenic. The question as to whether this abnormality in reaction stems from the basic weakness of character, or is a consequence of drug usage, is best studied when drug hunger is relieved. Patients on the methadone maintenance program, blockaded against the euphorigenic action of heroin, turn their energies to school work and jobs. . . . Their struggles to become self-supporting members of the community should impress the critics who had considered them self-indulgent when drug-hungry addicts. When drug hunger is blocked without production of narcotic effects, the drug-seeking behavior ends.[105]

Dole and Nyswander's groundbreaking work revolutionized the treatment of opioid addiction and improved the lives of many addicted individuals. Today, more than 250,000 Americans receive methadone maintenance therapy, also known as opioid agonist therapy, opioid replacement therapy, and opioid maintenance therapy. Studies done over many years in many countries, including Australia, China, France, Iran, Lithuania, Malaysia, Ukraine, and the United Kingdom, support the effectiveness of opioid agonist therapy.[106] A study in Norway, for example, demonstrated that individuals currently in treatment with methadone, compared to injection drug users not in treatment, have significantly fewer nonfatal overdoses, commit fewer thefts, report less drug dealing, and use less heroin.[107] Treatment for this population not only benefits the individual user but also contributes to the public good by reducing crime, HIV infection, hepatitis, and overall mortality, even when those receiving treatment are not able to achieve continuous drug abstinence.

Opioid agonist therapy is also cost-effective. A US study examining how opioid agonist therapy affects patterns of medical care, addiction medicine services, and costs from the health system perspective found that patients receiving opioid agonist therapy plus addiction counseling have significantly lower total health care costs than patients with little or no addiction treatment (mean health care costs with opioid agonist treatment = $13,578, versus mean health care costs with no addiction treatment = $31,055).[108]

Despite the wealth of evidence supporting its effectiveness, opioid agonist therapy is still controversial. Doctors giving patients an opioid to treat an opioid addiction seems counterintuitive. Other barriers to methadone treatment include having to show up at a methadone maintenance clinic daily, which is stigmatizing for many people. Also, methadone, especially when first initiating therapy, carries a high risk of accidental overdose.

Suboxone (buprenorphine-naloxone) is the only FDA-approved opioid agonist therapy besides methadone for opioid addiction. Suboxone first became available for the treatment of opioid addiction in the United States in 2002, after passage of the Drug Addiction Treatment Act (DATA) of 2000. The DATA 2000 allowed doctors for the first time in almost a century to prescribe an opioid for treatment of opioid addiction from an office-based practice. (Methadone for opioid addiction can only be prescribed from specialized methadone maintenance clinics. Only when methadone is prescribed for pain can it be prescribed in another facility.)* The 1914 Harrison Narcotics Tax Act had criminalized opioid addiction as well as the use of any opioid "for the sole purpose of maintenance."

Suboxone has important advantages over methadone. A month's

---

* The fact that methadone for the treatment of opioid addiction can only be given at a methadone maintenance clinic, and methadone for the treatment of pain can be dispensed from any doctor's office without any kind of special licensure required, is one of the enduring double standards in modern medical practice and another illustration of how addiction treatment is marginalized and stigmatized. Methadone prescribed in pill form for pain, not methadone from methadone maintenance clinics, has been a major contributor to the high opioid painkiller overdose death rates in the 1990s and 2000s.

supply can be obtained directly from a doctor's prescription, eliminating the need to attend a daily clinic. Suboxone has a ceiling effect on respiratory suppression, which means it does not have the same risk of accidental overdose due to respiratory suppression that is seen with methadone and other opioids. It binds and stimulates the opioid receptor as heroin, morphine, and methadone do, but it does not create the same kind of intense high users experience with other opioids. It decreases or blocks the effects of other opioids if taken at the same time.[109]

Denial

Denial, a common feature of addiction, also plays a role in the drug-seeking patient, and it has its own unique characteristics when it comes to prescription drug misuse. Denial is a defense mechanism that seeks to ignore some aspect of reality, because to acknowledge that reality in that moment would overwhelm the psyche. An acronym for denial among members of Alcoholics Anonymous is *"Don't Even k(N)ow I Am Lying,"* which captures the subtle internal dialogue drug-seeking patients have with themselves to justify their actions. In the context of drug-seeking patients, denial allows the addicted individual to rationalize compulsive drug seeking as help seeking: "I need this medication for my pain." If such patients were to get their drugs from the street or an illegal Internet pharmacy, they would be moving out of the patient role and into a more conspicuous "drug-addict" role, making it that much more difficult to preserve a patient identity and justify drug use on the grounds of recovery from illness or injury.

But drug-seeking patients are also motivated by an authentic belief in their illness narrative. They genuinely believe they are sick and need the medication to survive. In many instances, they truly are sick, with painful medical conditions that require treatment. Their belief in their need for certain medications has been bolstered by their previous experiences with doctors who also believe in their illness narrative and are willing to prescribe for them. Neither patients nor their doctors will easily or willingly unwind these narratives just because the medical establishment decides to change course in the way such patients are treated.

The Prisoner's Dilemma and Tit for Tat

Given that patients addicted to prescription drugs are physiologically driven to seek out and consume those drugs and will manipulate doctors to get them, and given that doctors are limited in their capacity to know which patients are benefitting from the drugs they prescribe and which are misusing or are addicted to them, doctors are caught in what behavioral economists call the prisoners' dilemma.

The prisoners' dilemma describes a situation in which mutual cooperation is advantageous, but one-sided betrayal is more advantageous to the one who betrays. The classic example usually put forth by economists is two criminals arrested for a crime and placed in solitary confinement with no ability to communicate. If both remain silent (mutual cooperation), both get parole. If each testifies against the other (mutual betrayal), both serve two years in prison. If one testifies against the other and one remains silent (one-sided betrayal), the one who testifies walks free, and the one who remains silent gets ten years.

A doctor prescribing potentially addictive drugs to a patient who is at risk to misuse or become addicted to them, which is virtually any patient, faces a prisoners' dilemma. If the patient takes the medication as prescribed (mutual cooperation), the patient's pain is treated and the doctor fulfills her mission as healer. If the patient takes the medication other than prescribed (misuse and one-sided betrayal), the patient gets what she wants (even if it's not what she needs), but the doctor has failed in her mission as healer. If the doctor refuses to treat the patient (one-sided betrayal the other way), the doctor is rid of a complex patient, but the patient loses access to care. Nothing in a doctor's training or education prepares her for the complexity of this kind of encounter.

Game theorist Robert Axelrod invited academic colleagues from all over the world to devise computer strategies to compete in an iterative prisoners' dilemma tournament. The programs that were entered varied greatly in complexity, aggressiveness, and capacity for forgiveness. Many competitors used Bayesian models and meta-analyses to try to predict future moves. With repeat encounters over a long period of time, each using different strategies, greedy strategists tended to do very poorly, while more altruistic strategists were more successful. (The nonretaliating strategy of "always cooperate" was also one of the least successful strategies, systematically exploited by "nasty" strategies.)[110]

The winning strategy in the tournament was contributed by Anatol Rapoport, who entered Tit for Tat, the simplest of any submission, containing only four lines of BASIC.[111] Tit for Tat begins with mutual cooperation, but once betrayal occurs, it is followed by retaliatory measures commensurate with the betrayal, a pattern that continues until mutual cooperation is reestablished.

Here's how Tit for Tat looks in the case of a prescription-misusing or addicted patient. First, the doctor agrees to treat the patient, and the patient agrees to comply with treatment, that is, take the controlled medication as prescribed (mutual cooperation). As long as the patient cooperates and takes the medication as agreed, the doctor continues to prescribe. However, once the patient betrays the doctor, for example, by visiting another doctor for a duplicate opioid prescription, the doctor immediately responds by giving the patient only a one-week rather than a four-week supply of the medication and insisting that the patient come in weekly for a month to get urine drug screens before each one-week refill. Note: the doctor does not verbally reprimand the patient and do nothing, the absence of retaliation. The doctor also does not fire the patient for betraying the contract—what game theorists call permanent retaliation. The doctor retaliates commensurate with the level of betrayal and stops retaliating once the patient course-corrects.

Although there are no studies exploring the use of Tit for Tat in the clinical scenario of the prescription drug-misusing patient, there are data from other populations of drug users implying its potential utility, at least as a short-term strategy, in the ongoing prescription drug epidemic. Those under criminal justice supervision (before trial, on probation, or on parole) are often drug tested at least once per week, but sometimes more often, with the sanction for a missed test or positive urine screen being one twenty-four-hour period in jail. These swift, targeted interventions, known as contingency management, have been shown to reduce drug use and promote abstinence. By contrast, harsh, nonspecific criminal sanctions for drug use or possession are generally not an effective deterrent.[106]

6

The Professional Patient

Illness as Identity and a Right to Be Compensated

With all the time Jim was spending seeking out doctors to get prescriptions, he was unable to go to work. He took a medical leave, which was extended with the promise that he could return to his job when he was able, a lucky scenario, and one not afforded many workers. Jim thought about applying for disability income from the federal government, but instead lived off of his considerable savings during this time. In *not* applying for disability, Jim may have inadvertently paved the way for his recovery. One of the factors that would ultimately propel him into addiction treatment was the need to go back to work to pay the bills. By contrast, many patients I see who are on disability become trapped in a situation in which maintaining their income means perpetuating their illness status, which both fuels prescription pill consumption and bars the way to addiction treatment.

Staying Sick as a Means of Survival

During a routine Wednesday morning outpatient clinic, Sally rolled into my office in her wheelchair, her service dog at her side, and began to elaborate at length on her various medications—Prozac and Zyprexa for mood, Klonopin and Ambien for sleep, Xanax for breakthrough anxiety, Lamictal for epilepsy, Requip for restless legs, oxycodone for pain, Vicodin for breakthrough pain, morphine for more breakthrough pain, Baclofen for muscle spasms, and Adderall for attention deficit disorder.

At age 29, Sally was receiving more medical care than most 85-year-olds.

Looking over her chart, I noticed that neurologists had never found an explanation for the "leg weakness" that confined her to a wheelchair, nor any definitive evidence of seizure. Outside of her own subjective endorsement of symptoms, there was no objective medical evidence to corroborate her diagnosis.

Moreover, her multiple medications were causing side effects, including obesity, gum disease, sexual dysfunction, diabetes, and addiction to painkillers and Xanax. Yet despite these medication-induced adverse medical consequences, with minimal relief of her original symptoms, Sally was not interested in changing her treatment. "I'm sick and I'm not getting any better, doctor. I've tried everything, and this is as good as it's going to get." My only utility to Sally was refilling her prescriptions and signing off on her disability paperwork so she could continue to receive $800 per month in Social Security Disability Income.

Sally represents a type of patient I see with increasing frequency: patients who visit a doctor's office not to recover from illness but to be validated in their identity as a person with an illness. They are afflicted by ailments of indeterminate validity, take multiple medications, often ten to twenty pills per day, and suffer adverse consequences from the very medical interventions meant to help them, including addiction to prescription drugs. Their medical charts are replete with phrases like "drug-seeking," "secondary gain," "noncompliance," "somatic," "early refill," and "medication overuse," all of which covertly communicate that their doctors are suspicious of their motives and overwhelmed by not knowing how to help them. Importantly, most of these patients are poor, undereducated, and reliant on federally funded disability as their primary source of income. In other words, they are professional patients.

Professional patients are not simply feigning illness; they are adopting social roles. Social roles are not created by individuals. They emerge organically in a given time and place, within a given society, an amalgam of cultural tropes, social norms, and economic incentives. Each social role comes with its own rights, obligations, and responsibilities. Writing in the latter half of the twentieth century, sociologist Talcott Parsons described "patients" and "doctors" as social roles within modern society. The primary responsibility of the patient, Parsons argued, is to "try to get well"; the primary responsibility of the doctor is to "minimize illness and disabilities."[112]

Although little more than sixty years have passed since Parsons's original writings on the social roles of patients and doctors, his ideas no longer apply to a growing segment of the patient population. Within the last three decades, a transformation has occurred in American society and medicine, such that patients are no longer necessarily obligated to get well, and doctors no longer necessarily obliged to minimize disability. Indeed, today staying sick has become a means of survival and keeping patients sick a new way of helping. Poor patients in particular are financially incentivized to be on disability.

Rising Disability Rolls

According to the work of economists David Autor and Mark Duggan in *The Growth in the Social Security Disability Rolls: A Fiscal Crisis Unfolding*, the number of adults receiving disability through Social Security Disability Insurance (SSDI) has increased almost twentyfold since 1957. In 1957, some 150,000 nonelderly adults were receiving disability payments through SSDI. SSDI is one of three major federally funded programs to financially support those who cannot work due to illness but who have paid Social Security taxes through prior employment. By the end of 1977, however, that number had risen to 2.8 million.[113] The two other large government-sponsored disability programs, Supplemental Security Income (SSI), for low income or indigent disabled persons, and Veterans Disability Compensation (VDC), for military personnel with service-connected disabilities, have likewise seen tremendous growth in the last several decades.

The largest recent increases in disability claims have been for mental illness and chronic pain disorders. In 1983, heart disease and cancer represented the largest fraction of disability insurance awards through SSDI. By 2003, mental disorders and musculoskeletal disorders (for example, back pain) constituted the largest fraction of disability insurance awards, 25 percent and 26 percent, respectively—approximately double their 1983 rates. Among children, diagnosed mental illness is the leading cause of SSI disability, a thirty-five-fold increase from two decades ago, far outdistancing physical disabilities like cerebral palsy or Down's syndrome. Among veterans, post-traumatic stress disorder (PTSD) is the most common mental health service-connected disability, with an increase of ~150 percent in disability benefits payments between the years 1999 and 2004, accounting for 21 percent of all benefit dollars paid through the VDC.[114] Paradoxically, overall health outcomes in adults between ages 50 and 64 have improved since 1984.

So why are more Americans than ever before applying for and receiving disability income? Autor and Duggan argue that disability programs have come to "function like a nonemployability insurance program for a subset of beneficiaries, rather than (primarily) as an insurance program for medical impairment" (87).[113] They note two major changes in Social Security disability policy in the last several decades which have contributed to this phenomenon.

First, starting in the early 1980s, the monetary value of Social Security disability insurance began steadily rising, especially for lower-income wage earners, making disability more attractive than available employment options. The 1996 welfare reform bill, which required states to reduce the numbers on welfare and report that reduction to the federal government, may also have provided an incentive to states to move poor people to the disabled category to improve the state's welfare numbers.

Second, in the mid-1980s congressional disability screening laws were revised to emphasize applicants' reported pain and distress and to deemphasize objective medical criteria. Subsequently, more and more claimants were filing for syndromes with few or no objective criteria, especially post-traumatic stress disorder and depression, but also physical illnesses that are difficult to validate with laboratory or imaging studies (such as chronic pain, multiple sclerosis, seizure disorders, chronic fatigue syndrome, late whiplash syndrome, fibromyalgia, myalgic encephalitis, chronic temporomandibular disorder, repetitive strain injury, sick building syndrome, Gulf War syndrome, etc.).

Poverty and lack of education are important determinants of who seeks disability, independent of illness status. In 2004, high school dropout males were five times as likely to receive SSDI disability payments as males with a college degree.[113] Vietnam veterans who are most likely to be on disability through the Veterans Disability Compensation program are not those with the most war-theater exposure or wartime injuries, but rather those with the lowest predicted earning potential, based on previous education level and skills.[115] Much of the recent increase in new PTSD claims by Vietnam veterans seeking disability is for conditions that were not evident on the battlefield, suggesting that their symptoms are as much a result of their life circumstance since being discharged from the military as to the military experience itself.[116] According to the US Census Bureau's figures for 2006, of the 40 million people in America who receive disability compensation, most are poor and undereducated.

The Complicity of Doctors and Health Care Institutions

Doctors and health care institutions are complicit in the medicalization of poverty that encourages the creation of professional patients. The doctor-patient interaction has in some instances been reduced to little more than a business arrangement, in which helping the patient secure income becomes the primary goal—likewise a financially rewarding proposition for hospitals and doctors.

For-profit firms called "eligibility service providers" are hired by hospitals to help uninsured patients apply for SSI benefits as a means of reducing the number of uninsured patients they have to treat. Disability is usually accompanied by automatic Medicaid benefits. Once patients have Medicaid, the hospital and clinics can be reimbursed through Medicaid for services rendered.[117]

Doctors commonly receive unsolicited mailings, encouraging them to fill out disability forms in exchange for cash. I received the following unsolicited e-mail in my inbox in 2014:

> Dear Doctor, Millions of Americans are out of work and the new phenomenon is that they are applying for State Disability Benefits once their unemployment benefits are exhausted. Did you know that Disability Determination Services pays approximately $175 for a 30 minute office visit? That's $2800 per day for a 16 patient load. We have the only software on the market designed to help you complete the Social Security Disability musculoskeletal exams and get it turned around in minutes. If you modify your practice to see State Disability clients just one day out of the week you would add $140,000 to your practice. You would net $136,000 after taking into account the cost of the software.

An early historical precedent for the financial incentives afforded doctors vis-à-vis the professional patient, can be traced to the late 1800s, when the inception of the railroads led to the establishment of insurance companies to compensate individuals harmed in railway accidents. Shortly thereafter, a problem called "railway spine" manifested, defined by a vague cluster of symptoms such as fatigue and nervousness in individuals who had experienced even very minor train jarring. Forensic psychiatrists, who had previously been confined to examining prison inmates, now were needed to evaluate cases of railway spine, and were of course compensated as well by the railroad insurance companies for this work. The number of cases of this condition rapidly proliferated, as did the number of doctors to treat it, illustrating that the success of railway spine as an accepted diagnosis was intimately related to the monetary benefit to both victims and healers.[118]

Professional Patients at Risk for Prescription Drug Addiction

Professional patients may be at increased risk of becoming addicted to prescription drugs because of greater exposure to these drugs.

The granting of disability has been shown to increase health care consumption, which in turn increases risk of exposure to prescription medications. The granting of disability for PTSD in veterans, for example, is followed by an increase in the use of both mental health and medical services, with medical visits increasing by as much as 30 percent and mental health visits by as much as 50 percent. In those denied compensation, mental health visits decline by as much as 50 percent in the postclaim period.[114]

Professional patients are treated for conditions that rely on each patient's subjective endorsement of symptoms: chronic pain, depression, attention deficit disorder, post-traumatic stress disorder, and so on. These types of disorders are treated with medications that acutely improve subjective feelings of pain, anxiety, dysphoria, fatigue, and cognitive impairment. The medications that target pain, feeling, and thinking are also the medications with the highest potential for misuse, dependence, and addiction: opioid painkillers, sedative hypnotics, and stimulants.

Patients seeking disability may have to take medications to validate their claims status. In a December 2010 issue of the *Boston Globe*, journalist Patricia Wen tells the story of an impoverished single mother living in the projects of Roxbury who applied for Supplemental Security Income for her three sons when she could no longer afford to pay her bills.[117] Her neighbors told her about the program and encouraged her to pursue it. She was initially reluctant to label her sons as having attention deficit disorder, preferring to view them as rambunctious; but the money—thousands of dollars per year and automatic Medicaid coverage—was eventually too good to pass up. Her first several rounds of applications were denied. Then friends and neighbors told her that her sons needed to be on stimulant medications like Ritalin or Adderall to get disability approval. She found a doctor who agreed to put her sons on a stimulant. The next time she applied for disability, her claim was successful.

Doctors are more likely to prescribe opioids and other addictive medications to patients on Medicaid,[119] many of whom are receiving disability payments. People receiving Medicaid are prescribed painkillers at twice the rate of non-Medicaid patients, and they die from prescription overdoses at six times the rate. New York State Medicaid enrollees are more likely to die from opioid painkiller poisonings than those not enrolled in Medicaid: deaths per 100,000 among New York State residents not enrolled in Medicaid increased from 0.73 in 2003 to 2.82 in 2012. Deaths among New York State residents enrolled in Medicaid increased from 1.57 to 8.31 over the same period.[119] Veterans with PTSD, 94 percent of whom have VDC disability for PTSD,[120] are prescribed opioids for chronic pain at a higher rate than those not in that category.[121]

The reasons for higher rates of controlled prescription drug prescribing, especially opioids, in the Medicaid and PTSD-veterans populations are unclear, but many doctors I spoke with reported feeling they have little else to offer these patients, who often lack access to behavioral treatments, physical therapy, acupuncture, or other alternatives to prescription drugs in the treatment of chronic pain and mental health disorders.

Furthermore, many patients receiving disability payments have independent risk factors for addiction, including poverty, unemployment, social distress, and lack of alternative rewards.[122] New disability applicants cannot qualify for disability based on their addictive disorder alone. A congressional law passed in 1996 disqualified SSDI claimants with addiction, terminating about 130,000 beneficiaries. Two-thirds of those claimants requalified for disability under a different disorder,[113] mostly chronic pain disorders, setting them up for addiction to prescription painkillers.

The Victim Narrative and Illness as Identity

Professional patients, in adopting the sick role, are vulnerable to developing an illness identity and a victim narrative, thereby increasing their dependence on doctors and prescription drugs and decreasing their likelihood of getting treatment for addiction.

In telling her story, Sally used borrowed language and medical jargon ("my PTSD," "my fibromyalgia," "my depression"). She gave a recitation of trauma and diseases that lacked the richness and detail that typically distinguishes one individual's life story from another's. Her use of the possessive pronoun was not merely convenient syntax but also a way of communicating that illness had become her identity. She saw herself as perpetually victimized by forces beyond her control and yet wholly dependent on others for recompense. This created in her an attitude of resentment and entitlement in equal measure, and influenced her perception that others misused and maligned her, even when the circumstances and facts argued against it.

Joseph Davis articulates in the journal *Social Problems*, "Gaining public sympathy and help for those putatively injured requires establishing their moral goodness, as persons innocent of any responsibility or fault for the harm they suffered" (530).[123] Fassin and Rechtman write in their book *The Empire of Trauma: An Inquiry into the Condition of Victimhood*, that "trauma is not simply the cause of suffering that is being treated, it is also a resource than can be used to support a right" (10).[118]

Over the last thirty years, illness has become identity and a victim narrative commonplace. The medical and social sciences are partly responsible for this trend. They have legitimized the categories of illness which provide the foundation for new identities. The Canadian philosopher Ian Hacking, in his article "Making Up People," argues that our culture creates people who didn't exist before. According to Hacking, this process occurs first by counting people with a certain trait or characteristic through the application of biostatistics to social sciences, then quantifying those characteristics (as in the *Diagnostic and Statistical Manual of Mental Disorders*), then providing a putative scientific explanation for this new identity.

Hacking gives as an example the fact that autism was a rare developmental disorder in 1973, occurring at a rate of 4.5 per 10,000 children, whereas today the autism spectrum disorders—for example, "Asperger's"—occur at a rate of 57 per 10,000, spurring the debate about whether the disorder has increased, detection has increased, or our expanded definition has increased diagnosis, or all of the above. Whichever way, says Hacking, the social and medical sciences have created people with new biologized identities which provide a way "to be a person, to experience oneself, to live in society."[124]

The adoption of illness identities is also driven by the breakdown of traditional social roles. Illness provides a way to define the self in a rapidly changing and increasingly fragmented world. Furthermore, ill persons today are lionized as heroes because they fight a battle against overwhelming physical forces. In a world in which the struggle for basic survival (food, clothing, shelter) has become largely irrelevant for most Americans, the ill person is among the last of the great warriors.

Illness identities furthermore offer a chance for community. Patient advocacy groups declare national disease-related holidays, hold educational conferences, produce media, publish literature, and sponsor websites, all encouraging individuals to regard themselves as distinct and separate because of their illness. Patient advocacy groups, too, are often funded by the pharmaceutical industry. For example, CHADD, Children and Adults with Attention Deficit Hyperactivity Disorder, is a not-for-profit patient advocacy organization that receives 14 percent of its total revenue ($345,000) from pharmaceutical grants, including the makers of methylphenidate and amphetamine salts (stimulants).[125]

Illness as identity is not in all cases a bad thing; it can give people a sense of purpose and belonging and provide some relief from suffering in knowing they are not alone. An illness identity is less stigmatizing than other identities, for example, being unemployed. But when illness subsumes identity and provides the only roadmap for living, and when treatment involves the continual ingestion of controlled drugs, then addiction is not far behind. Furthermore, the victim narrative of the professional patient almost guarantees that the patient cannot get better. When an individual's survival becomes predicated on having a chronic and incurable illness, then that individual must stay ill.

A colleague with whom I shared care of a professional patient sent me this missive regarding our mutual patient:

> Pt arrived agitated and angry. Last week we had discussed her improvement and I noted that I thought she no longer met criteria for depression. Over the past week, she experienced panic at the thought that her disability status (and therefore livelihood) would be taken away if she no longer qualified for a depression diagnosis. In addition, she received two partial bills for psychiatry services and assumed she was being billed because she had improved or that her diagnosis had been taken away. Pt arrived today reporting suicidal ideation this past week and showed me photographs of her cluttered house to indicate how impaired her functioning remains.

My colleague, when she saw this patient again, worked to help her imagine a future in which she could be functional and working again. Her patient continued to be resistant to this idea.

A potential antidote to the victim narrative of the professional patient might be found in the so-called recovery movement, which encourages individuals to identify with their illness but not to be victims of it. Instead, it urges ill people to come together and use the healing power of the community to triumph over illness.

The recovery movement arises out of the tradition of Alcoholics Anonymous and other twelve-step self-help groups. One of the mechanisms by which AA helps people stop drinking is to give them a new narrative. The AA illness narrative teaches members that their intemperate substance use is caused by a disease, even going so far as to say that members are "allergic" to their drug of choice, thereby removing some of the shame associated with their past behavior. But the AA disease narrative of addiction is not a fatalistic one, however it may appear on the surface. In fact, one of the most important tenets of the AA philosophy is that members are responsible for their life choices. This truth is often misunderstood by critics of AA, who see the disease model and the Higher Power elements of the AA philosophy as an invalidation of individual will and choice. To the contrary, emblazoned on AA literature throughout the world are the three words "I am responsible." AA teachings thus embody a paradox: a disease narrative that speaks to inevitability, but not to helplessness; a spiritual journey that emphasizes reliance on a Higher Power, but not an abdication of personal choice or responsibility.

Disability as Safety Net or Social Harm?

I worked with Sally for more than a year to try to whittle down the number of medications she was on, particularly the addictive ones. I tried to establish an effective method of communication between myself and her six other doctors, and to move her on a path toward true wellness. I thought we were making some headway, but then Sally informed me that she had found yet another doctor, a sleep specialist, who diagnosed her with narcolepsy and recommended the highly addictive medication GHB, also known as the "date rape" drug for its ability to render recipients virtually unconscious for some period of time. Sally embraced her new diagnosis of narcolepsy like finding a long-lost friend. She was relieved. The sick role was what she knew. And when I told her I could not condone the addition of yet another potentially addictive medication to her regimen, she walked out of my office, and I never saw her again.

Frueh and colleagues write in the *American Journal of Public Health* that "disability policies require fundamental reform to create an effective, responsive, and flexible safety net. . . . We must ensure that . . . finite resources are not misallocated and do not foster invalidism."[120] Economists Autor and Duggan suggest specific ways to reform our current system.[126]

In the meantime, the sad plight of professional patients today can be aptly compared to the tragic plight of street beggars the world over, particularly those who maim themselves or their children to procure an income, a phenomenon seldom seen in modern America, but one that was quite common on the streets of nineteenth-century American cities and that still occurs in some countries today. Like street beggars, professional patients sacrifice their bodies to make a living, the crucial difference being that doctors play a role in maiming them, and the medium is addictive prescription drugs.

7

The Compassionate Doctor, the Narcissistic Injury, and the Primitive Defense

Jim continued to obtain enough opioid prescriptions from multiple doctors to feed his habit for approximately a year. Then one day he went to see one of his regular walk-in-clinic providers for a refill and was met by a physician who was so angry he refused even to let Jim be escorted back to an exam room. "I don't want to see you back in this clinic ever again!" he shouted, when he saw Jim's face. "Get out. Get out!"

What prompted this doctor's response?

Jim's insurance company used a tool called a Prescription Drug Monitoring Program (PDMP), which provides information on all the prescriptions for controlled medications a patient picks up at a pharmacy within a given time period (usually a year) and a given geographic region (usually within that state). These databases gather information collected from pharmacies by the Drug Enforcement Agency (DEA), including type of drug, strength and quantity of the drug, date the drug was picked up, pharmacy location, and which doctor prescribed it. The insurance company mailed this information to Jim's doctor, who saw his name among many other prescribers, all doling out opioid painkillers to Jim.

When Jim's doctor discovered that he was just one of many doctors giving Jim opioids, he became enraged, a demeanor at odds with what we usually consider to be appropriate for the compassionate healer. On a superficial level, Jim's doctor's reaction was understandable. Jim had lied to and manipulated him, and nobody likes being lied to. On the other hand, Jim had real pain and real addiction, and he needed medical help. To understand how a compassionate doctor could respond this way, let us spend some time looking closely at the psychology, background, and guiding principles of the average, well-intended doctor.

Who Is the Compassionate Doctor?

Doctors are by and large pleasers. They make it through the complex maze of schooling all the way to medical school by figuring out early on what other people want and providing it. They are temperamentally anxious, obsessional types, preferring structure and certainty to loose boundaries and uncertainty.

They are motivated by a higher calling. When they graduate from college, usually near or at the top of their class, they can choose to go into any number of professions, from business to law to computer science. They choose medicine, however, because they are looking for a chance to make a real difference in the most tangible sense, by saving lives and alleviating suffering.

Once in medical school, doctors are called upon to empathize with patients and imagine their suffering as their own, without judgment. They are socialized to believe their patients, without second-guessing the veracity of their stories. The relationship between doctor and patients is founded on an assumption of trust and mutual cooperation.

Once they enter practice, these perennial A-students are intensely invested in being the best doctors they can be. They are, in other words, narcissistically invested in being successful doctors. This is not to say that doctors are narcissists; narcissism is not the exclusive domain of pathological self-involvement. The psychoanalytic conception of narcissism leaves room for "healthy narcissism." Freud described early childhood self-involvement as a normal and healthy part of development. The psychoanalyst Heinz Kohut believed that when the narcissistic demands of early childhood are adequately met by available caregivers, then childhood narcissism evolves into healthy adult self-esteem.[127] The healthy narcissism of adulthood is what allows us to invest our energy and creativity into the things we care about to achieve success, however we define it, whether that activity is bird-watching, parenting, or doctoring.

So how do doctors define success? By mutually affectionate interactions with patients. These mutually affectionate interactions are often characterized by a patient's expression of gratitude. What balm to a doctor's soul when the patient says, "Thank-you, doctor, you have really helped me," or "Thank-you, doctor, I don't know what I would have done without you." More objective measures of doctoring success matter, too—a chemotherapy regimen that has eliminated a cancer, or a knee replacement that allows a patient to walk again. But for doctors working day in and day out treating patients, many of whom are chronically ill and will never get better but can only hope not to get worse, the most essential measure of success is a positive, trusting, mutually affectionate interrelationship.

At its most professionally satisfying, the interaction between doctor and patient can even approach the spiritual, or what philosopher and theologian Martin Buber called an "I and Thou" moment: "Man wishes to be confirmed in his being by man, and wishes to have a presence in the being of the other. . . . Secretly and bashfully he watches for a YES which allows him to be and which can come to him only from one human person to another."[128] These moments of deeply shared humanity, which thankfully occur often enough between doctor and patient, make all the years of schooling, all the exams, all the nights on call, all the petty bureaucratic demands (which seem to get only worse with each passing day) worthwhile.

When the Compassionate Doctor and the Drug-Seeking Patient Meet

When the compassionate doctor and the drug-seeking patient meet, what the doctor experiences is anxiety. Maybe not consciously, but there is anxiety nonetheless. If the doctor mistrusts the patient or questions the patient's story, then the doctor is not living up to the principles of empathy and compassion. If the doctor openly challenges the patient, she risks the mutually affectionate interaction that is key to measuring her day-to-day success as a "good doctor." On the other hand, if she doesn't challenge the drug-seeking patient, then she is also not living up to the ideal of the compassionate healer. In short, the doctor is stuck between a prescription and a hard place, and the result is anxiety.

What does the doctor do with this anxiety? She buries it by turning to primitive, largely unconscious defense mechanisms. First described by Freud, defense mechanisms are automatic, unconscious psychological maneuvers human beings employ to avoid having to cope with or even acknowledge uncomfortable emotions. The psychiatrist George Vaillant classified defense mechanisms into four levels, from pathological defenses such as denial, to immature defenses such as wishful thinking, to neurotic defenses such as rationalization, to mature defenses such as humor.[129] The important implication of Vaillant's classification is that we all employ unconscious defense mechanisms all the time to defend against all types of anxiety; and in times of acute distress, defenses mechanisms, even primitive ones, are adaptive. However, in our everyday lives, defense mechanisms tend to be maladaptive and should not be confused with coping strategies, which are adaptive and conscious. Typical defense mechanisms doctors use with drug-seeking patients include passive aggression, projection, splitting, and denial.

"Passive aggression" is defined as aggression toward others expressed indirectly or passively, most often through avoidance and procrastination. Examples include finding reasons to cancel visits with such patients, rounding quickly on them in the hospital, or not at all, writing extended refills to minimize contact, not returning their phone calls, etc.

"Projection" is attributing a moral or psychological deficiency in ourselves to another individual or group. Doctors often project the contempt they feel for themselves around lax prescribing onto their patients. It is easier for doctors to see patients as morally deficient than to acknowledge having abdicated their responsibilities to patients by prescribing medications that might be harming rather than helping them. In this scenario, the doctor thinks "What is wrong with this patient? Can't she get it together and take the medicine like she's supposed to?!" instead of "What is wrong with me, and with the system, that I would prescribe a medication I know is not helping?"

The "splitting" defense involves segregating experience into all good and all bad categories, with no room for ambiguity or ambivalence. Doctors typically engage in splitting by mentally segregating drug-seeking patients into the category of "bad patients" as distinct from "good patients." A good patient takes many forms depending on the doctor, but is often the patient who expresses gratitude, gets better, or can be seen quickly. Bad patients are those who threaten the doctor's sense of competence as healer or who trigger negative emotions, such as anxiety, impatience, or anger.

Of all the primitive defenses doctors employ against drug-seeking patients, the most common and insidious is probably denial. "Denial" is the refusal to accept a threatening reality by simply believing it doesn't exist. This includes refusing even to perceive or acknowledge certain truths, for example, that we are in the midst of a national prescription drug epidemic. For the past two decades, even very good doctors have ignored suspicious patterns of medication use, dispensed early refills, disregarded escalating doses, and failed to access data that would give them the information they need to make a more accurate assessment of current medication use, such as their state's prescription drug monitoring program (PDMP). Despite a major public health campaign to encourage doctors to register for and utilize their state's PDMP, only

35 percent of doctors practicing in the United States today access this resource.[130] Time constraints hinder doctors' ability and willingness to gain access to and utilize the database, but without checking the PDMP, responsible prescribing of controlled drugs in the modern health care system borders on impossible.

New legislation in some states mandates that doctors gain access to their state's PDMP. Some states have even gone further, requiring that doctors check the PDMP before writing a prescription for any scheduled medication.[131]

Narcissistic Rage, Retaliation, and Its Consequences

What happens when primitive defenses like denial no longer work, for example, when the prescription drug–monitoring database shows overt drug-seeking, and the doctor is forced to acknowledge that she has been supplying drugs to an individual who has been misusing them? At this point, the doctor is unmasked as nothing more than a gatekeeper of goods and services, or worse yet, a drug dealer, and she experiences a narcissistic injury. A narcissistic injury strikes at the heart of her sense of competence and self-esteem. It is extremely painful to experience, and the reaction is primordial, reflexive, and hostile. Jim's doctor's reaction—his unbridled rage and rejection of Jim—is a classic example of a narcissistic injury followed by narcissistic rage and retaliation. The idealized response, by contrast, is compassion and professionalism even in the face of these challenges.

Jim's doctor is not alone. In the last five years, the entire medical profession has experienced a narcissistic injury as a result of the media spotlight highlighting the harm done to patients from drugs obtained from doctors, tarnishing doctors' reputations and publicly shaming them. As a result, some doctors have not merely become more cautious about prescribing opioids to patients in pain but have gone so far as to refuse to treat pain, declaring it to be out of their scope of practice. These refusals have become so prevalent that drug-seeking patients have earned their own moniker, coined by Dr. Steven Passik: "opioid refugees." The term is apt, as one imagines these patients wandering from clinic to clinic trying to find a doctor to treat their pain. Furthermore, the rejection of these patients is not likely to be attributable to the stigma of addiction: doctors don't throw patients out for misusing alcohol, smoking cigarettes, or even being addicted to heroin. It is the doctors' complicity in the patient's addiction which triggers the narcissistic injury and the retaliatory response.

This kind of permanent retaliation has created more problems than it has solved. Some patients may be turning to illicit sources of opioids—namely, heroin—since doctors are no longer willing to prescribe for them. However, the relationship between doctors' prescribing patterns and the initiation of heroin use remains unclear.[132] What is apparent is that heroin use has increased since 2011, as have heroin-related overdose deaths.

Opioid Refugees

My patient Macy became an opioid refugee. I first met her in the pain clinic where I was asked to assess whether or not she had become addicted to prescription painkillers, and more importantly, what might be done for her if she had. When she first saw me, she was in her early twenties. I was just one stop in a very long road of doctors. As I came to know her, I realized that her story started with the story of her father, Mike. He was her primary caregiver when she became ill in her mid-teens.

Mike grew up poor in the 1980s in the drug-ridden neighborhood of East Oakland, which transitioned in a single generation from a mixed ethnic middle-class neighborhood to a predominantly poor black one, notorious for gang drug warfare. Mike was the youngest of five children, and every member of his family, except Mike and his oldest sister, was addicted to something.

As soon as Mike was old enough, he got out of East Oakland and started a family of his own. He was determined to give his kids a better life, as far away from drugs as possible. He and his young wife moved to a townhouse in Fremont, a middle-class community south of Oakland. They had two daughters: first Katherine, and then, seven years later, Macy came along. Their life was complete.

When Macy was a junior in high school, she began experiencing unbearable leg pain. Mike, to whom she had always been especially close, wasn't sure what to make of it and assumed it was growing pains, so did nothing. But a month later, Macy collapsed while playing volleyball at school and was rushed to the nearby emergency room. The doctors performed a number of tests and couldn't find anything wrong with her. Despite the absence of any pathology, they gave her intravenous morphine to treat the pain and sent her home. Two weeks later Macy was back in the emergency room with the same pain. More tests revealed an unusual mass on her diaphragm and on her ovary. The doctors worried it was cancer, and they switched from intravenous morphine to intravenous Dilaudid, and she was admitted for surgery to remove the tumors.

As it turned out, the mass on her ovary was a teratoma, a benign growth of no consequence. The mass on her diaphragm was a bit of lung tissue, also benign, the resection of which was more involved and required yet another hospitalization and more surgery. The doctors hoped the removal of the masses would eliminate Macy's pain, although a relationship between the masses and her pain had never been clearly established. In the meantime, she was given intravenous morphine, Dilaudid, and hydrocodone, all potent opioids with addictive potential, during and after each surgery. Altogether, Macy was hospitalized for two months, October and November of 2010, and barely remembers any of it because she was so altered by prescription painkillers.

At no point in the course of Macy's medical procedures was the risk of opioid addiction discussed. Nor was Macy's family history of addiction considered relevant. When Macy's various surgeries were complete, her doctors declared that she should be pain free. Despite having received heavy doses of opioids daily in the hospital for two consecutive months, Macy was sent home without a single pill. For the next six weeks, she experienced excruciating opioid withdrawal—nausea, vomiting, fever, chills—as well as unbearable muscle and bone pain throughout her body, even worse than the original leg pain.

In the grips of opioid withdrawal, Macy would lie on the floor screaming and crying out. Her parents, unsure what else to do, took her back to the local emergency room every few days, where she was given the opioids her body craved and promptly discharged again. Sometimes the doctors would readmit her to the hospital and give her intravenous morphine to control her pain, then discharge her again without opioids, follow-up, or any semblance of a treatment plan. Between 2012 and 2014, Macy's parents took her back and forth to the emergency room in an endless cycle of despair and frustration. The doctors never seemed able to tell them what was wrong with Macy, or how to help her, except for writing more opioid prescriptions.

Then, in 2014, on one of the emergency room visits, the doctor came out of the room and said to Mike with barely veiled hostility, "Is your kid on drugs?" He was implying street drugs like heroin, not the painkillers Macy's doctors were prescribing, although chemically speaking there is almost no difference between the two. Would his reaction have been the same if Macy were white instead of black?

"No," said Mike, without a moment's hesitation.

"How do you know?" challenged the doctor.

"I know because I know my daughter, and because we're with her all the time, and because she's not hanging out with other people doing drugs."

"Your daughter is a drug addict," the doctor said. "Don't come back here for pain medicine again."

Mike said nothing. He was without words. He gathered Macy up in his arms and drove her home. When he got her there, she lay on the floor, moaning and crying out.

"Give her some pain pills," he said to his wife and daughter Katherine, who were looking on helplessly.

"They're all gone," said his wife, a pleading look in her eyes.

"Dammit," Mike shouted. He wanted to shut his eyes and make it all go away. Then he made a decision.

"That's it," he said, grabbing his car keys. "If those doctors won't help her, I will." Without another word, he left the house and got in his car. He headed back to the old neighborhood, silent tears streaming down his cheeks. He still had some old friends who sold drugs. He would find them and buy some Percocet, or some heroin if he had to. That would stop Macy's pain.

As Mike was driving, a memory from his childhood intruded on his thoughts. He was crouched at the base of the chimney in his childhood home, tracing the outline of the inner brickwork with his chubby fingers, looking for the hole between bricks where the mortar had long ago crumbled away. He felt the divot and shoved his fingers inside, hoping for the crinkle of plastic. He found it. He pinched his fingers to get a hold of the bag and slowly pulled it out.

"Mommy, Mommy," Mike called, "I found one!"

He ran to the kitchen holding the plastic bag in front of him, the little blue and red pills bouncing around inside of it.

His mother was cleaning the kitchen, tired after working one of the many jobs she had over the years—housecleaning, cooking at a local diner, working the line at the Del Monte Cannery, forklift driving. Mike was her fifth child, with a different father than the rest, her child of that no-good drunk she sent away the day Mikey was born, knowing in her heart he wasn't going to be the father her son needed. She dried her hands on her apron and folded the little boy in her arms.

"You found one, so you get a dollar from me," she told him, "just like I promised."

She reached inside her purse and handed him a dollar bill.

"Now you listen to me," she said, kneeling down and looking him in the eye, "I don't want you ever doing those drugs like your brother and sister. It's no good, no good."

"I won't Mama," he said, "I promise. I don't ever want to make you cry."

As if waking from a dream, Mike took the next exit off the freeway, turned the car around, and drove home again. When he got home, he bundled the still crying Macy back into his car and took her to a different hospital emergency room. After hours of waiting, the doctor finally came. Mike turned to him and said, "This is my daughter Macy, and she has terrible pain all over her body which no one can understand. She is also addicted to pain pills, and doctors made her that way, so don't turn your back on her. Don't judge her. Help her."

This new doctor, perhaps humbled by Mike's desperate admission, took Macy in and admitted her to the hospital, using the occasion to get her a treatment plan that included assessment and treatment for addiction, which had never previously been suggested or offered and which is how she eventually ended up with me.

Once in addiction treatment, Macy's problems did not magically disappear, but with time, patience, courage, and effort, Macy made her way slowly to a better place, with decreased pain, improved function, a job, and plans for the future, which Macy also deserves.

A Doctor's Obligation

We doctors and other health care professionals have a heightened obligation to patients who have become addicted because of the treatment we have provided. We simply cannot turn these patients away to fend for themselves. Many of them become addicted without even realizing what has happened to them. Most of them have serious medical conditions that warrant medical attention, in addition to a life-threatening iatrogenic problem. Yet we shun them. Refusing to treat patients whom we discover are misusing prescription drugs is not an ethical or helpful response to the prescription drug epidemic.

8

Pill Mills and the Toyota-ization
of Medicine

After being exposed by his insurance company as a "doctor shopper," Jim was forced to travel farther to clinics he had never used before and to pay cash for his medical visit, usually about $80 per visit, as well as for his medication at the pharmacy.

One day, Jim went to a new clinic he had never visited before, farther from home, in a thriving part of Silicon Valley. He walked up to the receptionist desk to make his payment, but to his surprise, the receptionist, a fashionably dressed woman in her twenties, informed him that he would pay after his visit with the doctor, not before. That was unusual. In Jim's experience, these walk-in clinics always wanted their money upfront. Jim mentally shrugged and took a seat in the waiting area.

He found himself in a typical doctor's waiting room—chairs, a table with old magazines on it, a plastic rubber tree in the corner. Only one other patient was waiting with him: a thin middle-aged woman who looked worn and anxious, unable to sit still in her seat. Jim immediately recognized the signs of opioid withdrawal. When she told Jim she was there for pain, Jim started to relax. He was in the right place. The receptionist, who apparently also doubled as the nurse, called the woman's name and ushered her through a heavy door. The woman came back out less than five minutes later with a prescription in hand. Jim saw this too as a good sign. This doctor didn't mess around.

The receptionist-nurse escorted Jim to an examination room and took his vitals. His blood pressure and heart rate were both elevated, because his supply of opioid medication had started to run low, and he was in mild opioid withdrawal. The nurse noted his vitals on a piece of paper and left him in the room to wait for the doctor.

The doctor, a man about Jim's age, came into the room. He was wearing a suit, not a white coat. He was talking on the cell phone, apparently angry about a business deal gone awry. Jim remembers him saying "We shouldn't have sold that stock." The doctor didn't acknowledge Jim immediately, but instead paced in front of him, still angrily talking on the phone. This was not usual doctor behavior for Jim, and he got a little nervous. When the phone call ended, the doctor put his phone into his pants pocket, turned to Jim, and said,

"How can I help you?"

This was more like it. Jim launched into his usual routine. But instead of his story eliciting the questions and empathic murmurs he was used to, this doctor just stared at Jim and said nothing. He did not read the discharge summary Jim was trying to hand to him; he declined even to take it in his hand. Only when Jim held up his left arm to show off his PICC line did the doctor finally respond, but not in the way Jim had expected. The doctor reached out and dismantled the bandages around the PICC line, as if checking to see that the catheter was really inserted into his vein and not a dummy catheter made to look like a real one. Once he had presumably satisfied himself that it wasn't a fake, he didn't bother to reapply the dislodged bandages but left them in disarray.

Jim said, "Um, do you think you could at least put on a new bandage?"

The doctor didn't respond. He looked at Jim knowingly and said, "For pain, it's $200."

"Huh?" said Jim. He wasn't following.

"I'll give you thirty Norco, but the visit is $200 for treating pain."

Awareness dawned on Jim. This wasn't a medical visit, it was pure and simple a business transaction. "No way," he said. "No way am I paying $200. The usual fee is $80." But he wanted, he needed those pills. "I'll give you $100 and that's it."

"$200," said the doctor.

"I'm not going to let you screw me," said Jim, and got up to walk out, his limp gone, the cane hanging loosely from his hand.

"Okay. $150," said the doctor, when Jim had gotten as far as the door.

Jim stopped and imagined what the rest of the day would look like for him if he didn't get those pills. Most likely he'd spend it in the bathroom, spilling the contents of his gut from both ends. He turned to face the man waiting by the exam table, and then swallowing what was left of his pride, he fumbled for his wallet, pulled out $150, and stretched out his hand. He was going to make the man come to him. The doctor walked over to Jim, took the money, and then took out his prescription pad. He wrote a prescription for Jim for a month's supply of Norco.

The receptionist didn't even look up as Jim walked out the door.

Later Jim would reflect, "Hunting down those drugs is horrible. You're craving them, and you're on edge because you're withdrawing, and then you have to scam some doctor, and that's a lot of work."

Jim's encounter with the drug dealer pretending to be a doctor was the moment he realized he had become a drug addict pretending to be a patient.

Corrupt Doctors and Pill Mills

The doctor who demanded cash in return for writing Jim an opioid prescription was indeed a drug dealer, although he had "MD" behind his name. He was not alone. Doctors more interested in money than in the well-being of their patients took advantage of the rising demand for opioid painkillers in the 1990s and 2000s as a way to get rich quick. Certain areas of the country were hit worse than others. Florida became an epicenter for ethically compromised and frankly illegal exchanges of prescriptions for cash between doctors and patients. In 2010 alone, manufacturers shipped enough oxycodone pills to Florida for every state resident to have thirty-four pills, that is, 650 million oxycodone pills.[133] In 2011, Florida boasted 856 pain clinics, many of which became known as "pill mills"—places "patients" could go and almost be guaranteed a prescription for an opioid.

Since 2011, following a law-enforcement crackdown on pill mills, the situation has improved. In 2013, the number of oxycodone pills shipped to Florida dropped below 313 million, the number of pain clinics dropped to 367, and opioid overdose deaths declined.[133]

To hear of doctors who unequivocally abdicate their ethical and professional responsibilities to their patients for secondary gain is a source of shame for all doctors. Yet are the rest of us so very different? All of health care has become overwhelmed by a hucksteresque opportunism, in which making a buck is the driving force behind practicing medicine. Even those of us who want to help find ourselves trapped in a bureaucratic maze of maximizing profit. The enormous pressures on doctors today to prescribe pills, perform procedures, and please patients, all within a disjointed medical bureaucracy and all with an eye on the bottom line, has contributed to the current prescription drug epidemic.

The Industrialization of Modern Medical Care

The increasingly industrial-scale, capitalistic approach to medicine was brought home to me one day in May of 2014, when I received the following invitation: "Please join us for a Kaizen on frequent visitors to the emergency room." I had no idea what "Kaizen" meant, although the writer of the e-mail seemed to assume this was universal knowledge.

Kaizen, I soon learned from Wikipedia, is Japanese for "change for the better." The Kaizen Method was famously adopted by the Toyota automobile company, encouraging workers on the assembly line to stop the moving production line if they identify any abnormality of production parts. Workers are also encouraged to suggest improvements to resolve the abnormality. Kaizen goals include "gauging measurements against requirements," "innovating to meet requirements," "increasing productivity," and "standardizing how to improve operations."[134]

The assembly line in a Toyota factory today is not much different from Ford's assembly line of the early 1900s. Workers are assigned to one specific production task at a specific station. The car arrives at the station, and the worker performs the specified task over and over again on each car that comes by. Expertise is measured by the workers' ability to "meet requirements." It would not be advantageous for a worker to decide one day to turn the screw left instead of turning it right, or to use yellow paint when the car is meant to be blue.[135]

Doctors today work in integrated health care systems. During the 1990s and 2000s, there was a mass migration of doctors out of private practice and into managed care organizations. Seventy percent of US physician practices were physician-owned in 2002. By 2008, more than half of US physician practices were owned and operated by hospitals or integrated health delivery systems, and that number just continues to rise.[136] The reasons for this shift included new payment structures and care models that have made it difficult for private practice to remain a viable option. Also, the younger generations of doctors, an increasing number of whom are women, are invested in preserving a work-life balance, and hospital employment makes it possible to have more flexible hours and protected off duty time.

The migration of doctors into integrated health care systems (hospital factories) has transformed medical treatment. Doctors work much less autonomously. Treatment options are often dictated by hospital administrators, Joint Commission (see chapter 4) guidelines, and third-party payers (health insurance companies). Like assembly-line workers, doctors are expected to "gauge measurements against requirements," "innovate to meet requirements," and "increase productivity."

No longer are doctors and patients alone in the exam room. They are accompanied by a host of invisible partners with demands that may have little to do with treating illness: Patient Relations stands gazing into the mirror, a patient satisfaction survey on a clipboard in her hand; Billing is standing on the scale, the numbers on display never far from his mind; Disability Claims sits with one leg in a cast, propped on the empty chair; The Joint Commission is digging through a file cabinet, a magnifying glass in hand; Private Insurance is occupying the chair intended for the patient, distracted and encumbered by a stack of prior authorization forms; the Centers for Medicare and Medicaid Services, morbidly obese, is leaning precariously on the edge of the exam table; Big Pharma hides in the corner, just out of sight, confidently spinning a drug company pen; the State Medical Board is hovering behind the doctor, looking stern and unyielding; and two lawyers, the hospital's Legal Counsel and the patient's Lawyer, are facing off, fists raised, ready to do battle. Time personified is there, ticking steadily, reminding the doctor that time is short and other patients are waiting.

The impact of this transformation on health care delivery, and its contribution to the prescription drug epidemic, cannot be underestimated. I receive monthly billing statements informing me whether or not I am meeting the clinical billing requirements set for me by my employer. They come as an e-mail complete with pie charts, graphs, and tables. Whereas I used to worry mostly about how best to treat my patients, I now spend time worrying about my billing targets and what I can do to change my practice patterns to meet them. When I rise above the line graph of my expected quota, I feel a surge of triumph, even a little surge of dopamine. When I dip below, I feel anxious about job security.

To more efficiently meet the billing quota ("innovate to meet requirements"), doctors do the math. If a psychiatrist provides psychotherapy (that is, spends time talking to the patient) for fifty minutes, he or she generates 2.79 Relative Value Units (RVUs). RVUs are the number assigned by Medicare and adopted by many other third-party payers to gauge the monetary value of a medical visit or intervention. At 2.79 RVUs, the hospital can charge $300. As a point of comparison, a screening colonoscopy (in which the doctor inserts a camera into the anus and up the gastrointestinal tract to look for disease) takes about 13.5 minutes and generates 15 RVUs, for a monetary value of $500.[137] Hence, a gastroenterologist (doctors who do colonoscopies) can theoretically generate five times what a psychiatrist doing psychotherapy can in the same amount of time.

But if a psychiatrist writes a prescription for a patient (a service called "medication management"), doing away with talk therapy and spending as little as a few minutes with a patient, he or she can bill a minimum of $230 for this service and, more importantly, can see many more patients per unit time. It is no wonder, then, that a whole generation of psychiatrists now calls themselves "psychopharmacologists," doing nothing more than prescribing psychotropic drugs.

The pressure to see more patients per unit time and to bill more per patient pervades all of medicine, encouraging doctors to continue to prescribe drugs. A family medicine doctor admitted to cherishing the patients who only need a quick refill: "Those are my easiest patients. They are scheduled for ten minutes, but if I give them what they want, they're out in five. Then there's hope I can catch up and get home at night." Most doctors are not mercenaries. They care about their patients and want what is best for them. But the pressures to get patients in and out quickly can be overwhelming.

Susie, a young emergency room doctor, finished her residency in emergency medicine and then opted for an additional year of training in addiction medicine. She wanted more experience treating patients with addiction because she had witnessed so many patients coming through the emergency room with serious alcohol and drug problems, including prescription drugs.

After completing a one-year fellowship in addiction medicine, Susie took a job in 2014 as an emergency room physician in a Bay Area hospital, where she continues to work today. She gets no base salary, no hourly salary, no retirement, and no benefits, including no health insurance. She pays for her health insurance separately through a private insurer. Health insurance costs her $800 per month. Although she is technically an employee of the hospital, she gets paid like an independent contractor. She makes 22 percent of what she bills. If she bills $7,000 in an eleven-hour shift, she makes $1,540. The more she bills each patient, the more money she makes.

"Whether I spend a lot of time or a little time with one patient," Susie said, "I get paid only for what I bill. If the crux of my interaction with patients is a conversation, I lose dollars, because talking doesn't pay."

When Susie encounters patients whom she suspects are misusing, diverting, or addicted to prescription drugs, she tries to take a little more time to talk with them about her concerns and looks at the prescription drug–monitoring database to assess the number of prescribers and types of prescription for controlled drugs they've obtained in the last year.

"But a lot of the time it's easier not to put up a fight and just give them the drug they want."

When Susie slows down to take more time for her patients, not only does she personally make less money but her corporate boss makes less money as well. Susie has been strongly advised to improve her numbers. One trusted colleague, someone Susie considers to be a "good doctor," told her to "just give them what they want and get them out the door." Susie's job represents an extreme form of the incentive-based compensation packages that many hospitals and health care delivery systems are moving toward.

If she could do it all over again, would Susie still practice medicine?

"I like people. I like helping people. If I could go back, I think I'd still do medicine. But the practice of medicine is so different from what

I thought it would be. I'm not someone who has ever been focused on money, but I am getting more focused on money now."

Patient Satisfaction: A Measure of Good Care?

The use of patient satisfaction surveys in health care is another example of the corporatization of medicine, and it has contributed to the prescription drug epidemic.

The idea of using surveys to assess patients' satisfaction with their medical care began in the 1980s. The rationale was based on a handful of studies showing that patients who are better satisfied with their care are more likely to be compliant with treatment and return to the same provider or facility the next time they need treatment.[138] "Treatment compliance"—doing what the doctor says—and "continuity of care"— seeing the same doctor over time—theoretically lead to improved patient outcomes. They are also good for the financial security of doctors, clinics, and hospitals.

One of the earliest organizations to turn health care surveys into a profitable business was Press Ganey Associates, founded in 1985 by Dr. Irwin Press, PhD, an anthropologist, and Dr. Rod Ganey, PhD, a statistician. On its website, Press Ganey describes what it does as "driving targeted performance improvement." The website goes on to state that "to improve the patient experience, health care providers must first be able to see and understand the complex relationships between satisfaction, clinical, safety and financial measures. Press Ganey's unique suite of solutions gives every patient the opportunity to be heard, integrating their voices with these distinct data streams and seamlessly weaving together millions of patient touch points."[139]

Patient-satisfaction surveys coincided with a larger "patient-centered care" movement in medicine, advocating for the patient to be viewed as the central figure in health care services. Today, many health care systems ask patients to fill out written or computerized surveys, rating their impressions of their doctors or the treatment they've received.

Although patient satisfaction surveys may be useful tools for improving certain aspects of health care, access, cost, and convenience, there is little or no evidence that patient satisfaction leads to improved medical outcomes, and some evidence to suggest that it may in fact lead to worse medical outcomes. In a study published in 2012 in the *Archives of Internal Medicine*, higher patient satisfaction was associated with higher consumption of health care services, higher prescription drug use, and increased mortality.[140]

Patient satisfaction is tightly linked to expectation, and when a doctor-patient interaction involves a "bad surprise," defined as care that is contrary to what was expected or goes against social norms, then patients are more likely to express dissatisfaction.[141] Nonetheless, good doctoring involves being willing to tell patients things they might not want to hear, such as concerns about substance misuse or addiction, or the need to withhold certain treatments because the likelihood of harm is too great.

The persistent use of patient satisfaction surveys, despite the lack of evidence to support their contribution to good care, and emerging evidence to suggest they may be linked to worse care, is rooted in financial incentives. Patient satisfaction has become, in many health care institutions, a "quality measure." A quality measure is one of the ways hospitals are rated by organizations like The Joint Commission and then ranked one against the other. This is not just a measure of pride but is also tied to financial reimbursement from third-party payers like the Centers for Medicare and Medicaid Services (CMS). CMS (federally funded health insurance for the poor, elderly, and disabled) collects data regarding patient satisfaction through the use of the Hospital Consumer Assessment of Healthcare Providers and Systems (HCAHPS) survey. The HCAHPS survey queries a random sample of adult patients two days to six weeks after discharge from the hospital and asks them about their hospital experience. A typical question on the survey is: "How often did the hospital staff do everything they could to help you with your pain?" In one year, HCAHPS collects hundreds of patient surveys from each hospital it reimburses. Scores on the HCAHPS survey can impact how much CMS is willing to reimburse the hospital for its services. Lower patient satisfaction means lower reimbursement. One emergency room that was struggling with low patient satisfaction scores implemented a policy of Vicodin "goodie bags" for each patient on discharge.[142]

For individual doctors, poor ratings on patient satisfaction surveys is a source of professional shame and, in some settings, can hinder professional advancement. My 11-year-old son was doing his homework on the computer, when for some reason he decided to google my name. One of the sites that came up was a doctor-ranking website with an evaluation of my professional abilities. My son called me into his room and said, "Mom, is this you?"

I looked at the site and, after taking a few moments to figure out what it was, realized that this particular patient, who called himself "Corey"—I don't remember him or even know if this is his real name—gave me one out of four stars. I don't believe zero stars was an option or I'm sure he would have given me zero. He wrote in the comments section: "Really wish I had seen this site's reviews before making an appointment with this physician." (There were in fact no other negative reviews on the site, which made this statement rather inexplicable.) "She provides the kind of care that will make you wish you had never sought help in the first place. Wrong diagnosis. Wrong medication. In some cases this can be terrible. Seek help from someone else."

I was flooded with shame, enhanced by the fact that my own son had found such a negative review on the Internet. Who else might have seen it? Perhaps I had told Corey I wouldn't refill a medication he was expecting to get. Perhaps with the next patient, I would just fill it. One pain medicine doctor I spoke with admitted that he had prescribed medications to patients he knew were misusing and addicted to them for the sole reason of avoiding that patient going onto Yelp and giving him a bad rating.

Practicing with Blinders On—Not Toyota after All?

Good communication between doctors today is essential to good care. Most patients have more than one doctor taking care of them, or they change doctors frequently due to insurance changes and other provisions of the managed care environment. Each doctor is busy prescribing the pills he or she believes will treat the patient, while other doctors are prescribing other pills. It is entirely commonplace to encounter a patient who is getting a stimulant from a psychiatrist for attention deficit disorder, an opioid painkiller from a pain doctor for fibromyalgia, and a benzodiazepine from a primary care doctor for sleep.

One of the promises of integrated health care systems, and their integrated electronic medical records, is that it will be easier for doctors to communicate with one another, so the right hand knows what the left hand is prescribing. Unfortunately, antiquated privacy laws, namely, a code of federal regulations known as "42CFR Part 2," prevents doctors from sharing information about patients with substance use disorders unless that patient gives the doctor written permission to do so.

42CFR Part 2 was originally conceived in 1972 as part of the Drug Abuse Prevention, Treatment, and Rehabilitation Act to encourage individuals with addictive disorders to seek treatment. This federal regulation was important, effective, and compassionate jurisprudence at a time when police enforcement was known to raid methadone maintenance clinics and arrest individuals seeking help if they tested positive for illegal drugs. Thirty years ago, 42CFR Part 2 was vital to protecting the rights of individuals with addiction and ensuring their access to addiction treatment.

Transposed to the current day, however, especially with our reliance on electronic medical records to coordinate and consolidate medi-

cal care, the same statute impedes the integration of addiction treat
ment into the larger health care system. As stated in a *New England
Journal of Medicine* commentary, these regulations "frustrate accountable care organizations and health information exchanges, since their
elaborate consent requirements make it difficult or impossible to share
patient data related to substance use disorders. As a result, many organizations exclude such information from their systems, undercutting
efforts to improve care and efficiency."[143]

The Centers for Medicare and Medicaid Services must redact all
records containing substance use treatment information of Medicare
recipients, about 20 percent of the Medicare population, when sharing patients' data with various accountable care organizations to fa
cilitate care coordination. Since 2015, half of the states in the United
States have Medicaid Health Homes, which serve millions of people,
especially those with mental illness and addiction. Prevalence of alcohol and opioid use disorders among Medicaid Health Home recipients
hovers around 80 percent. When clinicians gather via conference calls
to discuss individual patients to coordinate and optimize their care, behavioral health professionals must hang up when clinical substance use
issues are discussed.

A doctor working inside a large managed health care organization
described a patient of hers who suffered dire consequences as a result
of 42CFR Part 2. The patient was a high-functioning college professor
who drank on average a bottle of wine every night, more on weekends.
She was admitted to the medical unit of the hospital within the same
health care organization where she was being treated for her alcohol
use problems, but the doctors responsible for her medical admission did
not have access to the records describing her alcohol use. On admission
to the hospital, the patient herself may have minimized her use, presumably out of shame, or perhaps her doctors failed to ask her about it,
assuming a successful college professor could not also be an alcoholic.
Either way, several days into her hospital stay, the patient developed
fulminant life-threatening alcohol withdrawal, an experience she sur-

vived, but not without complications. She developed Wernicke's encephalopathy and Korsakoff's dementia as a result of belatedly identified alcohol withdrawal. In other words, she incurred irreversible brain damage because her treating doctors did not know that she was at risk to go into alcohol withdrawal, and by the time they realized what was happening, it was too late. Although 42 CFR Part 2 is waived in cases of emergencies, lack of timely access to a patient's substance use history in the electronic medical record, particularly during a medical crisis, limits the doctor's ability to provide the best care.

42 CFR Part 2 as it currently stands has contributed to the prescription drug epidemic by making it difficult if not impossible for doctors to tell other doctors whether a patient is misusing or is addicted to the medications they are prescribing. The result is doctors working at cross-purposes, with addiction specialists trying to get patients off a medication, while other doctors put them back on.

Doctors as Baristas

The current prescription drug epidemic is not the result of a small population of deviant doctors willfully harming patients,[144] although those doctors exist. Rather, it is the result of a large population of well-intended doctors working in health care factories that prioritize through-put of body parts on an assembly line over whole-patient health. The result is overprescribing, which is faster and better reimbursed than educating or empathizing with patients. Pills that are addictive are particularly likely to be overprescribed because they provide patient-customers with short-term satisfaction and a proxy for human attachment—but not necessarily improved health. When autonomy is truncated and professional status is linked to earning power and patient satisfaction surveys, doctors are vulnerable to objectifying patients as commodities rather than seeing them as people. Patients are vulnerable to utilizing doctors as nothing more than a source of drugs.

A San Francisco Emergency Department nurse was riding a public bus to work in 2012 when she overheard the following conversation between two women also riding the bus.

"What should we do today?" said the first.

"Not sure," said the second.

"Well, we could go to Starbuck's—or we could go to the emergency room."

They thought about it for a moment. Neither was in any apparent medical distress. "Let's go to the emergency room."

And so it was decided.

We have arrived at an era when going to the emergency room for a shot of Dilaudid (a highly potent opioid painkiller) or a few milligrams of Klonopin (a benzodiazepine sedative) is pursued by some as casually as ordering a shot of espresso. This scenario is the fault, not of the individuals who seek out substances for nonmedical use, but of a system that has allowed such a pursuit to be possible.

9

Addiction, the Disease Insurance Companies Still Won't Pay Doctors to Treat

When Jim first walked through my office door in 2013, he said, "Doc, I've got terrible pain, but I'm also addicted to painkillers, and right now my addiction is worse than my pain." His savings were gone, and his stamina for manipulating ever-shadier doctors had run out. He briefly considered getting heroin from a dealer, but he couldn't reconcile that behavior with his view of himself in the world. Heroin in particular represented a line he wasn't willing to cross (in contrast to the younger generation, for whom there often is no line).

Jim was unusual in acknowledging both problems. Many patients who become addicted to prescription drugs in a clinical setting are more reluctant to accept the idea that addiction has taken hold in their lives. With a narrative shaped in part by Alcoholics Anonymous, Jim already had a framework for understanding what had happened to him.

The obstacle to his treatment was not his lack of insight into the need for treatment. Indeed, contrary to popular belief that all addicted people are in denial about their addiction, many people with drug and alcohol use problems are well aware of their problem and desperate for treatment but can't get it because their insurance company won't pay for it, and they don't have the resources to pay for it themselves. (Private residential rehabilitation for addiction can cost upward of $50,000 per month.)

I prescribed Suboxone for Jim's opioid addiction and referred him for individual and group psychotherapy focused on addiction recovery. I also urged him to renew his commitment to AA and be honest with his AA sponsor about his addiction to prescription painkillers. Jim was more than willing to follow my treatment recommendations. The problem? I couldn't get his insurance company to agree to pay for it.

They first refused to approve the seven-day Suboxone prescription unless I filled out three pages of paperwork justifying "medical necessity." Meanwhile Jim was experiencing painful opioid withdrawal, having stopped using all opioid painkillers in anticipation of starting on Suboxone. I filled out the paperwork and faxed it to the insurance company, only to have it denied again because Jim had "chronic pain," and Suboxone was not FDA-approved for chronic pain. By this time I was on the phone yelling at some hapless insurance company representative, demanding to speak to his supervisor. "My patient has chronic pain *and* an opioid use disorder," I said through gritted teeth, "I am prescribing the Suboxone for his opioid use disorder, and if you don't approve this medication today, I will go to my local newspaper and expose you for denying much needed medical care."

They approved it, but the whole process required three days of back-and-forth dithering, hours of my time away from clinical care, and raging on the phone at someone I'd never met, not to mention the suffering Jim endured at home vomiting in his bathroom. Suboxone is tightly regulated, as it should be, because, as an opioid, it is potentially addictive. But had I written a prescription for an opioid painkiller—like Vicodin, Fentanyl, or OxyContin—Jim could have picked it up in the same hour. Barriers to Suboxone prescribing stem not from its addictive potential but rather from the consistent discrimination within the US health care system, and on the part of insurance companies, against patients seeking treatment for addiction.

A Brief History of the Disease Model of Addiction

The fight to get addiction recognized as a bona fide illness within the US health care system, which coincides with getting insurance companies to pay for its treatment, has been a long and often losing battle. Almost two hundred years ago Dr. Benjamin Rush published *An Inquiry into the Effects of Ardent Spirits upon the Human Body and Mind: With an Account of the Means of Preventing, and of the Remedies for Curing Them* (1819),[145] in which he argued that chronic drunkenness is a biological disease, a radical belief for its time. Most of his contemporaries still viewed excessive and problematic substance use as a moral failing, a sin. Dr. Rush called for the creation of "sober houses," places where "confirmed drunkards" could receive treatment. It wasn't until 1864 that the New York State Inebriate Asylum was opened in Binghamptom, New York, the first of its kind in the country.[146]

Today, addiction affects 16 percent of the US population, about 40 million people, far exceeding the number of people afflicted with heart disease (27 million), diabetes (26 million), or cancer (19 million). Disease burden due to addiction exceeds half a trillion dollars annually. Yet in 2010, only 1 percent of the total health care budget went to treating addiction.[147]

Even shifting public opinion on the cause of addiction has not managed to revolutionize the medical approach. A survey conducted by the National Center on Addiction and Substance Abuse (CASA) at Columbia University found that two-thirds of Americans now believe that genetics and biological factors play a role in the development of addiction, while a third continue to view addiction as a lack of will power.[147]

Compounding the problem, doctors are not educated in the treatment of addiction. Only 20–30 percent of primary care physicians feel "very prepared" to detect risky substance use, yet 80 percent feel "very prepared" to tackle hypertension or diabetes.[147] Even psychiatrists are poorly trained in screening and treating substance use disorders, and they often turn away patients with addiction. Among practicing doctors, less than 1 percent identify as addiction medicine specialists.[147]

Oddly, insurance companies have long been willing to provide expensive, long-term treatment for other chronic illnesses, for example, diabetes and kidney disease—including kidney dialysis, an expensive and protracted intervention. Even other complex mental health issues are better reimbursed than addiction treatment. Most insurance companies will now pay for gender reassignment surgery for individuals diagnosed with gender identity disorder, but they won't pay for emergent inpatient treatment for someone in acute opioid withdrawal.

Yet we know that with medical treatment, addiction behaves very similarly to other chronic illnesses with a behavioral component, such as type II diabetes (behaviors related to diet), including similar rates of compliance with treatment, remission, and relapse.[148] Individuals who actively engage in treatment for addiction have, on average, a 50 percent recovery rate,[106] which is on par with response rates for other mental health conditions, such as depression and schizophrenia, and at odds with what many people assume about addiction treatment—that it is hopeless. These data lend support to the argument that addiction can and should be managed within the health care system.

The passage of the Paul Wellstone and Pete Domenici Mental Health Parity and Addiction Equity Act (MHPAEA), signed into law in 2008, requires group health plans that offer mental health or substance use benefits to offer them at parity with medical and surgical benefits. The passage of the Affordable Care Act expands this protection to an additional estimated 62 million Americans. Yet insurance companies still do not reimburse for addiction treatment on a par with other medical illnesses, finding loopholes and work-arounds to deny care. There continues to be widespread discrimination in health plans against those with mental health or substance use disorders.

As long as the US health care system ignores addiction, it will be burdened with paying for the costly treatment of the downstream medical consequences of addiction, never getting to the root cause, and millions of Americans will continue to suffer. For every dollar the federal and state governments spend on addiction, ninety-five cents goes toward treating the medical consequences of addiction, and only two cents goes toward addiction prevention and treatment.[147] Prescription drug misuse and addiction is one of these many downstream consequences.

My patient Diana's life story is illustrative of the serious health consequences that ensue when a patient is treated in a health care system that does not teach or reimburse its doctors to recognize and treat addiction. Diana's story also exemplifies the chronic, relapsing, and remitting nature of addiction.

The Many Faces of Addiction

When Diana was just two-and-a-half years old, her mother was pushing her in the stroller down the aisle at Mervyn's department store when she saw a set of clown-face hair clips and decided she had to have them. She reached out to grab them, but her mother stayed her hand. Diana's mother had always been particular about what Diana wore, and she was not inclined to buy the clown clips.

In response to being denied what she wanted, Diana did not make a pouty face, whine, or cry. She screamed. She screamed again and again, with such intensity that people shopping in the aisle raised their heads in alarm. When they looked in the direction of the screams, they saw a pretty little girl sitting in a stroller, her head thrown back, her face in a distorted grimace, her legs kicking out at the air, and her mother, panicked and helpless in the face of her daughter's ferocious desire.[23–26]

Her mother hurried her out of the store and wrestled her into the car seat, Diana wailing and arching her back in protest all the while. Two hours after they arrived home, Diana was still screaming when her mother called her husband in desperation, asking him to come home from work and help her. When Diana's father arrived home, he put Diana, still crying, into his car, and drove for hours. This would be the first of many such drives to calm Diana down. Finally, Diana cried herself to sleep. When her father arrived back home, he gently transferred Diana from the car to her bed. As he was tucking her in, he noticed her little fist tightly gripping an object. He gently peeled back her fingers, one by one, careful not to wake her. There, in Diana's hand, were the clown-face hair clips.

From very early in her life, whatever emotions Diana experienced, she experienced with above-average intensity, chronicity, and duration, and she seemed literally incapable at times of moving past it. She also demonstrated a reflexive response to her in-the-moment desires, acting on those desires with such willfulness that she was unable to logically weigh the pros and cons of her behavior.

When Diana was 11 years old, her uncle called her "chubby"—just an innocent observation, made in passing—but she couldn't stop thinking about it, and kept comparing her budding, early adolescent body to the images of perfection she saw in fashion magazines. She was determined to get thin, but didn't want to deprive herself of the foods she liked to eat. Then she had an idea.

She sat in the dark, alone, at the top of the stairs, waiting for her parents and her older brother to go to sleep. It was midnight before her parents' bedroom light finally went out. She slipped downstairs, taking the steps one at a time, careful not to make a sound. She opened the refrigerator, the light from inside cutting across the darkness of the room. She took out the pasta dish with the creamy clam sauce, the one she had allowed herself only a few bites of at dinner. She ate it right from the serving dish, quickly, taking in three or four regular-size portions at once, until her belly felt too full to continue. She didn't worry though, because in her mind the calories wouldn't count. Less than five minutes later she was in her bathroom upstairs, behind a locked door, leaning over the toilet with her fingers down her throat.

Diana was 14 years old when her parents discovered her behavior, and by then she was making herself vomit every day, sometimes more than once a day. They moved into high gear, getting her a doctor, a counselor, a nutritionist. She did individual therapy, family therapy, group therapy. Her parents carefully monitored everything she ate. But even with all that intervention, it was hard for Diana to stop. Even she was surprised by how hard it was. She had long ago achieved the body she wanted, so for her, it was no longer about being thin. Instead, she found herself craving the release of tension that making herself vomit gave her. Sometimes she would binge and purge twice in a row, in order to extend the feeling. Years later, she would reflect, "A lot like my heroin addiction, bulimia was that same pattern of having this secret space that no one else knows about where you do this disgusting activity. Once you're doing it, once you're in it, you lose the meaning of why."

For decades the field of psychiatry has conceptualized bulimia nervosa as an eating disorder, defined by the ingestion of large amounts of food followed by purging that food, most commonly through self-induced vomiting. More recently, however, clinicians and scientists are comparing bulimia to addiction. Thirty to 50 percent of individuals with bulimia have an active drug or alcohol use disorder, compared with approximately 9–15 percent in the general population, and up to 35 percent of individuals who have an alcohol or drug use disorder also have an eating disorder, compared with about 1.6 percent in the general population. These high rates of co-occurrence provide some indirect evidence for a shared disease pathway.[149] Even more compelling is how the specific eating patterns seen in bulimia are particularly addictive and differentiate bulimia from eating disorders such as anorexia. Bingeing on food, particularly foods high in sugar, releases dopamine in the brain's reward pathway, similar to the mechanism of action of drugs of abuse.[150] The vomiting that follows acutely increases endorphins, the body's own heroin, to augment the increased extracellular dopamine.[151]

In 1995, when Diana turned 15, her parents sent her to one of the most elite private high schools in Silicon Valley. Her bulimia was improving, and they were determined that her future would be bright. Diana remembers spending most of her first few weeks at school figuring out who the popular kids were and how to be a part of their group.

Like herself, many of her classmates were the children of aging hippies. "Fleetwood Mac's niece was there!" But unlike Diana, they were worldly in a way that was foreign to her. And they used drugs. In an effort to fit in, Diana began smoking cigarettes. They laughed when she choked on her first puff. From cigarettes she quickly progressed to alcohol and marijuana, providing another example of "neighborhood" as a risk factor for addiction, in particular exposure to drug use at school.

Alternative Rewards Reduce Substance Use

At age 16, Diana had an epiphany. She decided she wanted to be an artist. She made a conscious decision to cut back on alcohol and drugs, get a job, save her money, and go to art school. With this goal in mind, she graduated from high school at 17, rented an apartment in San Francisco, and went to a fashion institute. She had some early modest success, with her own art show, a publication in a San Francisco fashion magazine, and a nomination for a fashion photography award. Her drug and alcohol use during these years was intermittent.

Diana's ability to curtail drug and alcohol use during this time speaks to the importance of alternative rewards—including even the promise of future reward—when trying to limit substance use. As Charles Duhigg describes so well in his book *The Power of Habit*,[152] to change deeply ingrained behavior, the individual must find a way to substitute a new reward for the old reward. The same phenomenon holds true for rats. If you put a rat in a cage with nothing to do but press a lever for cocaine, it will develop all the major behavioral signs of cocaine addiction. However, if you add another lever the rat can press for a sugary drink, or a wheel the rat can run around on for fun, then the likelihood of that rat becoming addicted to cocaine is much less, and a rat who is already addicted to cocaine will use less cocaine.[153, 154] For Diana, the accolades she received from her artwork helped curb her substance use.

Heroin Chic

By the time Diana was 20, she was solidifying her identity as an artist, and she decided that the next step for her was to move to New York. With financial help from her parents, she moved to Manhattan. The late 1990s was the height of "heroin chic" in Manhattan, when scantily clad emaciated young women with dark rings under their eyes represented the pinnacle of beauty. Life-sized posters of Kate Moss, the "it-model" of the decade, papered the streets of all five boroughs of the city, often defaced with the words "feed me" scrawled across Kate's skeletal figure.

Diana, an uncommonly pretty girl, with long brown hair, big brown eyes, and delicate bones, fit right in. She worked as a model but tried to establish herself primarily as a fashion designer and photographer. With her looks, as well as the fact that she came from money, Diana quickly insinuated herself into the upper echelons of the New York fashion world. It didn't take her long to discover that drugs and alcohol were an inherent part of that world.

Diana spent hours, and sometimes days, planning what she would wear for an evening out. She might visit vintage shops, or create a "mood board," to generate ideas for an outfit. Her date, often an older man of means, would pick her up around 6 pm, and together they would go to New York's meat-packing district, the heart of the art scene, where blocks of art galleries hosted openings, followed inevitably by the after-party.

Every evening out would begin with alcohol, wine, or champagne served in tall fluted glasses passed around on trays. Diana drank eagerly. "If I saw David Bowie—or Mick Jagger, I wanted to be ready. I didn't want to be star-struck." For Diana, these evenings out were not just leisure; they were essential to her craft. She was there in part to find out what other people were doing and to generate ideas, digest them, and re-create them in another form. The ideas came not just from the art on the walls but also from the people she saw, the clothes, the gossip. The sense of urgency was palpable, and relentless.

Dinner didn't happen until after nine, and by then Diana was exhausted and not a little drunk. That's where cocaine came in. Diana remembers that getting cocaine at a party in Manhattan was as easy as ordering pizza. Someone would just call a number—everybody knew a number—and drugs would be delivered to the door. Diana prided herself on never being the one to order drugs or pay for them, something, she told herself, "only addicts did." They were always given to her as a gift. She would go into the bathroom and line the cocaine up in neat rows on the lid of the toilet seat. Kneeling down delicately, she would snort the lines, one nostril at a time. Again, the bathroom was a familiar sanctuary, which perhaps should have been a warning sign. Still, Diana was busy learning her craft and collaborating with other photographers and fashion designers. She could go days at a time without using any drugs. All that changed after she tried heroin for the first time.

It was 2001. Diana had just turned 21, and the specter of the Twin Towers bombing was still months away. She went to a friend's apartment to do a photo shoot. The friend was a model, and they often collaborated on projects. Her friend ordered heroin and had it delivered to the apartment. She put the soft white powder on the back of a CD case, snorted it, and offered Diana some. Diana snorted one-fifth of a line and felt its effects instantly. The first thing she noticed was that "the noise was gone." The cacophony of her New York City lifestyle was now only a distant hum. More importantly, the relentless muttering of her own inner voice, mostly telling her she was no good, was also silenced. It wasn't euphoria she felt as much as a sense of relief at not having to feel. She also felt nauseated and ran to the bathroom to vomit. After vomiting, her very next thought was a certainty that she would do heroin again. "It was magical."

Heroin possession and distribution is illegal in the United States, but heroin is readily available on the black market, sold as white or brownish powder mixed with powdered milk, starch, sugars, or quinine. "Black tar" heroin is sticky like roofing tar, mostly produced in Mexico, and predominates in markets west of the Mississippi, for example, in

California. The dark color results from the processing method, which leaves behind impurities. Black tar heroin must be dissolved, diluted, and injected into veins, muscles, or under the skin. In its pure form, heroin is a white powder with a bitter taste, usually from South America. It dominates US markets east of the Mississippi, for example, in New York. Pure heroin can be snorted and smoked as well as injected. Once heroin enters the brain, it is converted to morphine, leading to an immediate rush.

Since coming to New York City, Diana had bought no drugs for herself, but she immediately began buying heroin. Using just a little each day, she made her first $50 purchase last for two to three weeks. When she had used it all up, she experienced nausea, vomiting, diarrhea, and muscle cramps. She assumed she had the flu, not realizing that she was in opioid withdrawal. Within a few months, Diana had progressed to a $100 a day habit, and she started getting a reputation as a "junkie." Using drugs was accepted in New York's glamorous world of fashion, but being a junkie was not. When the Twin Towers fell on September 11, 2001, she was so busy fashioning a line of white powder on a clean glass surface that she hardly noticed.

By 2003 Diana's life had completely unraveled. Her career in fashion photography was nonexistent, many of her friends had abandoned her, and her money was gone. So she left New York for California, hoping that a change in location would allow her to start over again. She went to private rehabs in California, paid for by her parents. Her medical insurance covered nothing. Despite private treatment, she kept relapsing. At her lowest point, she was living in a seedy apartment in San Francisco, paying weekly rent from the money she earned as a stripper, using the leftover cash to support not just her heroin addiction but also the habit of the boyfriend living with her, whom she'd met on the street buying drugs.

Medical Complications of Addiction—a Revolving Door

In 2005, when Diana was 24 years old, she developed pustular nodules on her skin as a result of having injected heroin for four years. The nodules quickly transformed into large red swollen patches all over her body. She also had difficulty breathing. Her father rushed her to the emergency room.

Electronic medical records from Diana's first hospital admission describe her left arm as covered with "swollen, pustular vesicles . . . draining fluid" with areas of skin that felt as if there were "cobblestones underneath." Her right arm was afflicted, as was the base of her right thumb. On her right ankle, she had a 4 cm cyst filled with blood and pus. The inner side of her left calf had a 2 x 2 cm open wound draining bloody purulent fluid. A chest X-ray revealed pneumonia, with possible infected heart valves. Cultures of her wounds were positive for the bacteria Staphylococcus aureus, a particularly virulent form resistant to the antibiotic Methicillin, and therefore known as MRSA—Methicillin-resistant Staphylococcus aureus.

She was diagnosed with severe MRSA furunculosis, MRSA bacteremia, cellulitis, and skin abscesses. The differential diagnosis at the time of admission included rare immune deficiency syndromes such as Hyper IgE Syndrome and Job's Syndrome. It wasn't till days after admission that her doctors asked her about intravenous drug use, which, according to the medical record, she initially denied. Collateral information obtained from her parents led to documentation of a clear history of heroin addiction, including intravenous use.

The medical consequences of heroin use, in particular intravenous heroin use, are many, and depending on route of administration, include but are not limited to constipation, pneumonia, tuberculosis, damage to mucosal membranes from snorting, perforated nasal septum, scarred or collapsed veins, bacterial infections of blood vessels and heart valves, abscesses and other soft tissue infections, hepatitis, HIV, and accidental overdose by slowing heart rate and depressing respirations.

Diana's treatment, which saved her life, included six different intravenous antibiotics, surgical drainage of her abscesses, and multiple skin grafts. For pain control she was given a long-acting form of morphine sulfate (MS Contin), 90 mg three times a day, dissolvable oral morphine, 50 mg every two hours as needed for pain, and intravenous fentanyl (another potent opioid), 100 mcg prior to every dressing change, which occurred two to three times per day. Diana was in the hospital for weeks, and as a necessary condition of her treatment, her brain was bathed in opioids the entire time. At the time of discharge, Diana's doctors were in general agreement that her infection and ensuing medical problems were the downstream result of her intravenous drug habit. Despite this awareness, no part of her otherwise very thorough discharge planning involved any recommendation or referral to addiction treatment. In a system in which doctors are not educated to recognize addiction as a disease, or paid by insurance companies or other third-party payers to treat addiction, it is logical that Diana's doctors ignored it.

Diana was sent home with an intense regimen of medications and treatments for her wounds and residual infection. She had a peripherally inserted central catheter (PICC) in her arm so that she could continue to receive intravenous antibiotics even after discharge. She was given follow-up appointments at the infectious disease clinic, the hand clinic, the pain clinic, the immunology clinic, the primary care clinic, and twice daily appointments at the ambulatory care clinic to receive an infusion of Vancomycin (an antibiotic) and dressing changes. She continued to receive MS Contin 90 mg three times daily after discharge, as well as fast-acting dissolvable tablets of morphine 60 mg every two hours as needed for pain, and 90 mg of the same prior to dressing changes, which occurred twice daily.

In the months that followed Diana's first hospital admission, as her wounds began to heal, her doctors attempted to reduce the opioids she was taking for pain. Not surprisingly, every attempt to reduce her opioids was unsuccessful. In response to her inability to comply with their recommended reductions, Diana's doctors refused to prescribe opioids any longer. Diana went from a steady high dose of prescription opioids, supplied by her physicians, to zero. Diana, no stranger to opioid withdrawal at this point in her life, briefly considered using heroin again but was terrified of recurrent infection. Instead, she found another solution.

With the sustained-release morphine sulfate pills she had left, she took a small pair of scissors and scraped the time-release coating off of the outer portion of the pill. She crushed it with a mortar and pestle down to a fine powder. She mixed the powder with the saline she'd been given by the doctors to flush out her PICC line and injected it intravenously through the PICC line. By changing the route of administration, she was able to increase the bioavailability of the pills she had left and thereby extend her supply. Diana's story mirrors that of other injection drug users in the late 1990s early 2000s, who switched from IV heroin to prescription opioids with the increased availability of the latter.[155, 156]

Given the absence of medical treatment for her addictive disorder, it was no surprise that Diana was unable to stop using opioids. Data show that untreated opioid addiction is characterized by relapse, noncompliance with medical treatment, and increased morbidity and mortality.[148] For the next three months Diana continued shooting up dissolved MS Contin from her leftover stash. In January 2006, Diana's mother walked in on her shooting crushed morphine into her PICC line and called the police.

The police put Diana on a legal hold called a "51-50," which allows a doctor to admit an individual against his or her will to a psychiatric ward for observation and treatment for seventy-two hours. Admitted to the same hospital where she had received her original treatment, Diana was now on the psychiatric unit rather than the medical unit. On the psychiatric unit, more than six months after she had been admitted to the hospital for the first time, Diana was at last formally diagnosed in the electronic medical record as having a drug addiction, or in the language of the latest *Diagnostic and Statistical Manual of Mental Disorders* (5th ed.), an "opioid use disorder."[15]

Physicians seldom officially diagnose and document a substance use disorder in the electronic health records (EHRs), even when they agree that a substance use disorder exists. Electronic health records have primarily become a means of justifying billing to third-party payers, that is, Medicare, Medicaid, and private insurance companies, rather than a record for documenting illness and its treatment.[157] Since doctors don't get paid to treat addiction, there's no reason to put it in the record. Some doctors also fear that the label will stigmatize patients and compromise their future care. More often, however, it's the lack of information on patients' substance use in the medical record that compromises their care.

Diana entered a residential addiction treatment center after her discharge. This treatment center cost her family tens of thousands of dollars for a thirty-day stay. Fortunately, they were able to afford it. Her care in the treatment center, which included treatment with Suboxone, allowed her to stop using opioids in one form or another for the first time in many years.

Benzodiazepines—the Hidden Prescription Drug Epidemic

Diana began seeing a psychiatrist after she was discharged from the hospital in 2005. Her psychiatrist added one psychotropic medication after another—antidepressants, mood stabilizers, anxiolytics, hypnotics—until she was taking upward of fifteen pills each day. Despite the hospital recommendations not to resume any benzodiazepines or other potentially addictive sedative hypnotics, Diana's psychiatrist initiated her on a course of the benzodiazepine Valium.

The first benzodiazepine, Librium, was synthesized accidentally by Leo Sternbach in 1955 and then marketed for the treatment of anxiety and sleep disruption by the pharmaceutical giant Hoffmann La Roche in 1960. The market success of Librium inspired the company to create another benzodiazepine, which they did with the synthesis of Valium in 1963. Valium was a best-selling drug for La Roche, the first to reach $1 billion in sales, and became the most widely prescribed drug for anxiety in the world. It also captured the American imagination, memorialized in the 1966 Rolling Stones hit "Mother's Little Helper."

Today, doctors' prescriptions for benzodiazepines continue to rise, and are a major culprit in the epidemic of prescription overdose deaths plaguing this country. Nonetheless, benzodiazepines are relatively ignored in the national discussion on rising rates of addiction. Many doctors are prescribing benzodiazepines to help patients get off of opioid painkillers, without recognizing or understanding that benzodiazepines themselves are highly addictive.

Diana started at a low dose of Valium, only 10 mg daily, but progressed to 10 mg twice a day, and in the weeks that followed quickly escalated to more than 100 mg daily, all prescribed by her psychiatrist. She did not do well. She lived with one or the other of her parents, was not able to maintain any kind of consistent employment, and was not able to engage in any of the artistic endeavors that had previously sustained her. Her psychiatrist diagnosed her with bipolar disorder, which she never felt fit her issues but which legitimized the federally funded disability check she got every month, the multitude of psychotropic medications she was on, and the monthly private-pay appointments. Between 2005 and 2013, she was essentially an invalid.

Addicted to Being a Patient

When Diana first came to my clinic in 2013, she did not self-identify as a person with addiction. She hadn't used heroin in years. But she was on a dizzying list of psychotropic medications, including Xanax to calm her down, Ritalin to pump her up, Depakote to even her out, Prozac to make her happy, and Ambien to put her to sleep. She was also using "medical marijuana" two to three times a day. Despite all these medications, she was anxious, distractible, emotionally incontinent, depressed, and unable to sleep.

In retrospect, of that particular moment in her life when she was taking fifteen or more pills and smoking cigarettes and marijuana daily, Diana would say, "I lost my voice. I was like one of those Victorian women diagnosed with hysteria and given laudanum. My doctor even told me I was a hysteric. I'd stopped using heroin, but I was a drug addict as much as ever. When I finally told my doctor I wanted to get off all the drugs and move ahead with my life, he told me I couldn't. He told me I was too sick, and I'd be sick forever."

Diana was admitted to the voluntary psychiatric unit that week and taken off all psychotropic medications except Suboxone, the only medication that consistently improved her function. When she was discharged this time, she went to weekly group therapy sessions focused on addiction recovery. She got a part-time job caring for her maternal grandmother, who was struggling with end-stage Alzheimer's. Most importantly, she got her brain back. She could think again.

A year after being discharged from the hospital, life is not easy for Diana. She continues to struggle with wide mood fluctuations and fits of rage, directed at those who care about her most. But she is not using heroin or any other illicit drugs. She even quit smoking cigarettes and marijuana. Sitting in group therapy, wearing faded jeans and a peasant blouse, twisting her long thick hair, she said, "For years I was a heroin junkie, and then I became a patient junkie, addicted to prescription drugs as much as I was ever addicted to heroin—maybe worse. But I got tired of being a junkie, and I got tired of being a patient. I help take care of my Grandma now. She has Alzheimer's, and I do a lot of things for her, just like taking care of a little baby. My mom says I take even better care of her than she does." With that she stops twirling her hair for a moment and smiles. "I want to be well, and hold on to my dignity as long as I can. I can think again, and I'm doing art again, and that feels really good."

Diana's story, from the toddler who demanded clown hair clips, to the "heroin junkie," to the young woman taking a fistful of prescription pills every day, illustrates the chronic relapsing and remitting nature of addiction and thus the need for a chronic-care model to treat it. It also highlights the profound ignorance of doctors, including even psychiatrists, who are supposed to be experts in mental illness, when it comes to detecting, diagnosing, and treating addiction. Diana's story, and Jim's, demonstrates how parity still does not exist within the US health care system for the treatment and reimbursement of addictive disorders.

10

Stopping the Cycle of Compulsive Prescribing

Jim did well with treatment for almost a year, abstaining from opioid painkillers and other addictive substance use during that time. What precipitated his relapse in the end was nothing dramatic or even particularly memorable. His insurance changed. The cab company opted for a new health insurance plan for its workers, and that plan did not cover my clinic. Jim couldn't find an addiction specialist in-network with his new plan (there aren't many of us), so he started over with a new primary care doctor.

My last conversation with Jim was by phone in 2014, when I called him to check in.

"How's it going, Jim? How are you doing?"

"I'm okay, doctor. I think I'm okay. But I had to stop the Suboxone, because, you know, I couldn't find anyone to prescribe it. And then my new doctor, she put me back on Norco for my back pain."

"But did you tell her about your history?" I asked.

"I told her about the alcohol, but not, er, the pills . . ."

"Jim . . . why not?"

"Because I really think I can handle it this time, Doc. I really think

I can. And the Norco works better for my pain. Maybe I'm headed down the wrong road . . . I'm probably headed down the wrong road . . . but for right now, this is what I gotta do."

"Would you like me to call your new doctor and talk to her about your situation?"

"No, Doctor, thank-you, but that won't be necessary."

"Are you sure?"

"Yeah, I'm sure."

Awkward pause. "Okay Jim, take care of yourself. Let me know if . . . you know . . . later, I can help."

"I will, Doctor. I promise I will."

I've not heard from Jim since. Jim, wherever you are, I hope you're okay.

Despite Policy Changes, the Epidemic Rages On

Since the CDC first declared a state of emergency around prescription drug addiction and overdose deaths in 2011, much has been done at the federal, state, and local levels to target the problem. Naloxone, a medication that can counteract a lethal opioid overdose, has been approved by the FDA, and Good Samaritan laws in many states now give doctors the ability to prescribe naloxone to patients, their friends, family members, or anyone who might witness and seek to prevent an opioid overdose.[158] Prescription drug–monitoring databases, which allow a doctor to check all the prescriptions a patient has received for controlled substances, have been implemented or invigorated in every state.[131] Hospitals, emergency rooms, and clinics across the country have created policies to limit opioid prescribing. Educational campaigns and guidelines on safe opioid prescribing have been launched. New prescribing guidelines now warn doctors of the risk of addiction to opioid painkillers. (Most of the interventions have targeted opioid painkillers. By contrast, almost nothing has been done to curb the more silent epidemics of stimulant [Adderall] and sedative-hypnotic [Xanax] overprescribing, misuse, and addiction.)

Despite these interventions, the prescription drug problem continues. From 2000 to 2014, almost half a million Americans died from drug overdoses. Opioid overdose deaths, including opioid painkillers and heroin, were the biggest driver behind these deaths, reaching record levels in 2014, with a 14 percent increase in just one year.[159] More than 200 million prescriptions for opioid painkillers continue to be written by US doctors every year.

Indeed, the prescription drug epidemic is likely to continue for the foreseeable future unless we do more to target the unseen forces driving the epidemic. (Even public discussion of these unseen forces verges on political incorrectness.) Cultural narratives promote pills as quick fixes for pain. Corporations in cahoots with organized medicine misrepresent medical science to promote pill-taking. Medical disability hinges on patients taking pills and staying sick as a way to secure an income. A new medical bureaucracy is focused on the bottom line, favoring pills, procedures, and patient satisfaction over patients getting well. And disjointed medical care and antiquated privacy laws make it impossible for the right hand to know what the left hand is prescribing.

Interwoven through all of this is the complex interpersonal dynamic between doctors and patients, riddled with mutual deception, wishful thinking, wounded pride, and desperate attempts on both sides to pretend that a doctor's only mission is to heal and a patient's only mission to recover from illness.

Even when addiction is recognized by doctors and their patients, doctors don't know how to treat it, no infrastructure exists to provide that treatment, and insurance companies won't pay for it.

How Can We End This Cycle of Compulsive Prescribing?

There is an unspoken tension underlying the hidden forces driving the epidemic: doctors are increasingly asked to care for people with complex biopsychosocial problems (nature, nurture, and neighborhood) without also being given the tools, time, or resources to accomplish this task. A little over a century ago, caring for the poor, the home-less, the unemployed, and the addicted fell to religious organizations. With the secularization of society in the early 1900s and the medicaliza-tion of many aspects of everyday life in the latter half of the twentieth century, doctors are now responsible for many more aspects of their patients' lives than what has traditionally been thought of as "disease." But, like trying to fit a too-large foot into a too-narrow shoe, doctors must "pretend" that their patients' problems are purely medical in or-der to shoehorn them into our current industrialized, fee-for-service, assembly-line health care system.

In order to address this mismatch, we as a society must restruc-ture the health care system to openly acknowledge the new mandate for medicine to care not just for those with physical illness but also for those with mental illness, including addiction. We must build a medical infrastructure that targets the problems people have, not assigns them problems they don't have to justify services within the existing system.*

Complex mental and behavioral problems require long-term care and the healing that is borne of relationship and community. Their treatment demands seamless integration with the rest of medicine, not the marginalized status they currently hold. Medicine must once and for all embrace addiction as a disease, not because science argues for it, but because it is practical to do so. As long as the system continues to ostracize patients with addiction, especially while openly embrac-ing and aggressively treating disorders such as chronic pain, chronic fatigue, fibromyalgia, depression, attention deficit disorder, and so on, the prescription drug epidemic will continue, as will the suffering of millions of people with untreated addiction.

In order to accomplish this goal, addiction treatment needs to be taught at all levels of medical education. Currently addiction is a very small part of most medical school curricula and is absent from almost

---

* The alternative is to decide that the medical system is not the appropriate venue to target poverty, unemployment, isolation, family dysfunction, etc., and to create social services outside of medicine which can do it better.

all residency training programs, including many psychiatry residencies. Medicine is learned through a series of apprenticeships. Residency lays the foundation for how doctors will practice medicine for the rest of their lives. Until training in addiction medicine permeates medical school and residency, the physician workforce will remain unskilled. One way to do this is to link federal funds currently used to subsidize medical school and residency training programs to mandatory inclusion of addiction medicine content.

Newly created addiction medicine fellowships represent progress toward this goal. These are fellowships that offer in-depth training in addiction medicine open to any doctor who has completed a residency in any clinical medical specialty, from trauma surgeons to anesthesiologists to primary care doctors.[160] The addiction medicine fellowships should be expanded and given better funding, and residents should be encouraged to participate in them.

The expanding medical workforce, including nurse practitioners and physician assistants, who in many states function de facto as doctors, must also be trained in addiction medicine. An analysis of Medicare prescribers in 2013 determined which medical specialties, based on sheer volume, were prescribing the most opioid painkillers. Family medicine was first, with 15,312,091 prescriptions in one year, followed by internal medicine, with 12,785,839 prescriptions. Nurse practitioners were third, accounting for 4,081,282 prescriptions, and physician assistants were fourth, with 3,089,022 prescriptions.[144] We clearly cannot, nor should we, ignore this influential and growing cadre of health care professionals.

Addiction treatment must be delivered in a chronic care model that prioritizes the importance of the doctor-patient relationship and the therapeutic environment. Doctors must be reimbursed not only for prescribing medications but also for talking to and educating their patients. This requires more *time with patients* than doctors in most health care organizations are currently granted. Time with patients is the essential precursor for empathic listening, informed judgment, and the healing power of human connection. The question is how to accomplish this.

New Models for Care

In 2010 the Kaiser Permanente Medical Group in Northern California recognized that there were opportunities to improve care for their patients dealing with chronic pain. Each separate Kaiser facility was encouraged to develop new programs that might better serve patients and improve patient outcomes.

Karen Peters, a clinical psychologist working at Kaiser Santa Clara's Chemical Dependency and Rehabilitation Program, and Barbara Gawehn, a registered nurse working in Kaiser Santa Clara's Chronic Pain Program, got together as part of a larger team to reimagine what a better pain program would look like, and how they might accomplish it. Both Karen and Barb had already been working together at Kaiser as part of an opioid taper program, and they were well acquainted with the phenomena of prescription opioid misuse, tolerance, dependence, and addiction. They also noted that once the opioid taper was complete and acute withdrawal symptoms were over, the patients actually had less pain than they had while on opioids. Being off the drugs made their pain better.

Karen, Barb, and their team decided that their new pain program would use nonpharmacological methods to target pain. In order to do this, they believed patients would have to be off opioids and other mind-altering medications, including "medical marijuana," which might cloud their ability to learn the techniques they were planning to teach, including mindfulness meditation. Therefore, any patients entering their program would have to be willing to taper down and off opioids, a process the team would facilitate.

They realized such a program would necessitate daily visits, at least initially, to provide the necessary psychosocial support for patients in opioid withdrawal and struggling with pain without opioid painkillers.

They planned to administer all treatment, including psychotherapy and physical therapy, in groups, because building a supportive community between patients was at the heart of their new approach. As Karen said, "I knew in my gut that a therapeutic community would be the vehicle for change, would be the provider, in essence." This idea of the group itself as the vehicle for recovery is deeply rooted in the philosophy of Alcoholics Anonymous and other mutual-help recovery groups. The main difference here was that the providers would be integrated into the community and would practice the interventions alongside the patients.

The program they created, which got under way in 2011, is little changed from the program that continues to this day. In the first phase, which lasts three weeks, patients come every day. In the second phase, which lasts three weeks, they come three times a week. In the third and final phase, which lasts at least a year but can go on indefinitely if patients choose to continue, patients are offered a menu of activities up to three days a week. Every day the program begins with every provider, including the doctors and every patient in the room, participating together in a series of activities that serve to teach and heal patients and also to build community—mindfulness meditation, chi gong, yoga, educational seminars, cognitive behavioral therapy, Feldenkrais, and even physical therapy. By sharing a common experience, patients and providers together build a common language, one that serves to shape an illness narrative, the core of which is that they need to "retrain their nervous system" to find a different way to manage pain.

Kaiser Santa Clara has now shepherded hundreds of patients through its Pain Management Rehabilitation Program, with remarkable transformations in the individual lives of many who have participated. Patients who were nonfunctional due to pain and lived hour to hour anticipating their next pain pill are now free of opioids and other addictive drugs and reengaged in their lives. This program serves as a potential model for how to help patients heal from chronic biopsychosocial disorders, including addiction and chronic pain.

A Clarion Call for Change

Understanding and ending the prescription drug epidemic is vital for all of us—doctors, patients, and their loved ones. People are dying every day from the adverse medical consequences associated with prescription drugs. Even absent harm to patients, doctors have an ethical responsibility to prescribe safely and judiciously and to stop prescribing when the risks of the drug overpower any foreseeable benefit. Patients have a right to quality care, even if it's not the care they think they need. The most valuable commodity each doctor has is his or her relationship with the patient. It's time to rethink how medicine is delivered, in order to preserve this central truth. The prescription drug epidemic is a symptom of a faltering system, a clarion call for change, not just for patients who have become addicted to prescription drugs, but for all patients and the doctors who treat them.

References

1. *Results from the 2012 National Survey on Drug Use and Health: Summary of National Findings*. Rockville, MD: Substance Abuse and Mental Health Services Administration; 2013. NSDUH Series H-46, HHS Publication No. (SMA) 13-4795.

2. Paulozzi LJ, Jones CM, Mack K, Rudd R. Vital signs: overdoses of prescription opioid pain relievers—United States, 1999–2008. *MMWR Morb Mortal Wkly Rep.* 2011;60(43):1487–1492. http://www.cdc.gov/mmwr/preview/mmwrhtml/mm6043a4.htm?s_cid=mm6043a4_w.

3. Warner M, Chen LH, Makuc DM, Anderson RN, Minino AM. *Drug Poisoning Deaths in the United States, 1980–2008*. Hyattsville, MD: US Department of Health and Human Services, CDC; 2011. NCHS Data Brief No. 81.

4. Chen LH, Hedegaard H, Warner M. Rates of deaths from drug poisoning and drug poisoning involving opioid analgesics—United States, 1999–2013. *MMWR Morb Mortal Wkly Rep.* 2015;64(32). http://www.cdc.gov/mmwr/preview/mmwrhtml/mm6401a10.htm.

5. Hall AJ, Logan JE, Toblin RL, et al. Patterns of abuse among unintentional pharmaceutical overdose fatalities. *JAMA.* 2008;300(22):2613–2620. http://www.ncbi.nlm.nih.gov/entrez/query.fcgi?cmd=Retrieve&db=PubMed&dopt=Citation&list_uids=19066381.

6. Lader M. Benzodiazepines revisited—will we ever learn? *Addiction.* 2011;106(12):2086–2109. doi:10.1111/j.1360-0443.2011.03563.x.

7. Paulozzi LJ. Prescription drug overdoses: a review. *J Safety Res.* 2012;43(4):283–289.

8. Han B, Compton WM, Jones CM, Cai R. Nonmedical prescription opioid use and use disorders among adults aged 18 through 64 years in the United States, 2003–2013. *JAMA.* 2015;314:1468–1478.

9. *Drug Abuse Warning Network, 2011: National Estimates of Drug-Related Emergency Department Visits*. Rockville, MD: Substance Abuse and Mental Health Services Administration; 2013.

10. Schedules of controlled substances: placement of tramadol into schedule IV. *Drug Enforc Adm Dep Justice.* 2014:2014-15548-; DEA-351. http://www.deadiversion.usdoj.gov/fed_regs/rules/2014/fr0702.htm.

11. Lembke A. From self-medication to intoxication: time for a paradigm shift. *Addiction.* 2013;108(4):670–671. doi:10.1111/add.12028.

12. *Diagnostic and Statistical Manual of Mental Disorders*. 5th ed. Washington, DC: American Psychiatric Association; 2013.

13. Ries RK, Fiellin DA, Miller SC, Saitz R, eds. *The ASAM Principles of Addiction Medicine*. 5th ed. Philadelphia: Lippincot Williams and Wilkins; 2014.

14. Schultz W. Potential vulnerabilities of neuronal reward, risk, and decision mechanisms to addictive drugs. *Neuron*. 2011;69(4):603–617. doi:10.1016/j.neuron.2011.02.014.

15. Kauer JA, Malenka RC. Synaptic plasticity and addiction. *Nat Rev Neurosci*. 2007;8(11):844–858. doi:10.1038/nrn2234.

16. George O, Le Moal M, Koob GF. Allostasis and addiction: role of the dopamine and corticotropin-releasing factor systems. *Physiol Behav*. 2012; 106(1):58–64. doi:10.1016/j.physbeh.2011.11.004.

17. Wise R, Koob GF. The development and maintenance of drug addiction. *Neuropsychopharmacology*. 2014;39(2):254–262. doi:10.1038/npp.2013.261.

18. Peele S. Addiction as a cultural concept. *Ann New York Acad Sci*. 1990; 602:205–220.

19. Gureje O, Mavreas V, Vazquez-Barquero JL, Janca A. Problems related to alcohol use: a cross-cultural perspective. *Cult Med Psychiatry*. 1997;21(2):199–211. http://www.ncbi.nlm.nih.gov/pubmed/9248678.

20. Marshall M. *Beliefs, Behaviors, and Alcoholic Beverages: A Cross-Cultural Survey*. Ann Arbor, MI: University of Michigan Press; 1979:451–457.

21. Kendler KS, Ji J, Edwards AC, Ohlsson H, Sundquist J, Sundquist K. An extended Swedish national adoption study of alcohol use disorder. *JAMA Psychiatry*. 2015;0126. doi:10.1001/jamapsychiatry.2014.2138.

22. Fabbri C, Marsano A, Serretti A. Genetics of serotonin receptors and depression: state of the art. *Curr Drug Targets*. 2013;14(5):531–548. http://www.ncbi.nlm.nih.gov/pubmed/23547754.

23. Iacono WG, Malone SM, McGue M. Behavioral disinhibition and the development of early-onset addiction: common and specific influences. *Annu Rev Clin Psychol*. 2008;4:325–348. doi:10.1146/annurev.clinpsy.4.022007.141157.

24. Vrieze SI, Feng S, Miller MB, et al. Rare nonsynonymous exonic variants in addiction and behavioral disinhibition. *Biol Psychiatry*. 2013. doi:10.1016/j.biopsych.2013.08.027.

25. Hicks BM, Iacono WG, McGue M. Index of the transmissible common liability to addiction: heritability and prospective associations with substance abuse and related outcomes. *Drug Alcohol Depend*. 2012;123(suppl): S18–S23. doi:10.1016/j.drugalcdep.2011.12.017.

26. Acton GS. Measurement of impulsivity in a hierarchical model of personality traits: implications for substance use. *Subst Use Misuse*. 2003;38:67–83. doi:10.1081/JA-120016566.

27. Castellanos-Ryan N, O'Leary-Barrett M, Conrod PJ. Substance-use in childhood and adolescence: a brief overview of developmental processes and their clinical implications. *J Can Acad Child Adolesc Psychiatry*. 2013;22(1):41–46. http://www.ncbi.nlm.nih.gov/pubmed/23390432.

28. McGloin JM, Sullivan CJ, Thomas KJ. Peer influence and context: the inter-

dependence of friendship groups, schoolmates and network density in predicting substance use. *J Youth Adolesc.* 2014;43(9):1436–1452. doi:10.1007/s10964-014-0126-7.

29. Clark HK, Shamblen SR, Ringwalt CL, Hanley S. Predicting high risk adolescents' substance use over time: the role of parental monitoring. *J Prim Prev.* 2012;33:67–77. doi:10.1007/s10935-012-0266-z.

30. Dishion TJ, McMahon RJ. Parental monitoring and the prevention of child and adolescent problem behavior: a conceptual and empirical formulation. *Clin Child Fam Psychol Rev.* 1998;1:61–75. doi:10.1023/A:1021800432380.

31. Loveland-Cherry CJ. Family interventions to prevent substance abuse: children and adolescents. *Annu Rev Nurs Res.* 2000;18:195–218. http://www.ncbi.nlm.nih.gov/pubmed/10918937.

32. Broning S, Kumpfer K, Kruse K, et al. Selective prevention programs for children from substance-affected families: a comprehensive systematic review. *Subst Abuse Treat Prev Policy.* 2012;7:23. doi:10.1186/1747-597X-7-23.

33. Robins LN, Slobodyan S. Post-Vietnam heroin use and injection by returning US veterans: clues to preventing injection today. *Addiction.* 2003;98:1053–1060. doi:10.1046/j.1360-0443.2003.00436.x.

34. Paulozzi LJ, Mack KA, Hockenberry JM. Vital signs: variation among states in prescribing of opioid pain relievers and benzodiazepines—United States, 2012. *Morb Mortal Wkly Rep.* 2014;63(26):563–568. http://www.cdc.gov/mmwr/preview/mmwrhtml/mm6326a2.htm.

35. *Results from the 2012 National Survey on Drug Use and Health: Summary of National Findings.* Rockville, MD: Substance Abuse and Mental Health Services Administration; 2013.

36. McDonald DC, Carlson K, Izrael D. Geographic variation in opioid prescribing in the U.S. *J Pain.* 2012;13(10):988–996. doi:10.1016/j.jpain.2012.07.007.

37. Humphreys K. *Circles of Recovery: Self-Help Organizations for Addictions* (Edwards G, ed.). Cambridge: Cambridge University Press; 2004.

38. Project MATCH RG. Matching alcoholism treatments to client heterogeneity: Project MATCH posttreatment drinking outcomes. *J Stud Alcohol.* 1997;58:7–29.

39. Kelly JF, Hoeppner B, Stout RL, Pagano M. Determining the relative importance of the mechanisms of behavior change within Alcoholics Anonymous: a multiple mediator analysis. *Addiction.* 2012;107(2):289–299. doi:10.1111/j.1360-0443.2011.03593.x.

40. Sobell LC, Cunningham JA, Sobell MB. Recovery from alcohol problems with and without treatment: prevalence in two population surveys. *Am J Public Health.* 1996;86:966–972.

41. Steketee JD, Kalivas PW. Drug wanting: behavioral sensitization and relapse to drug-seeking behavior. *Pharmacol Rev.* 2011;63(2):348–365. doi:10.1124/pr.109.001933.

42. Nestler EJ. Is there a common molecular pathway for addiction? *Nat Neurosci.* 2005;8(11):1445–1449. doi:10.1038/nn1578.

43. Cadoni C, Pisanu A, Solinas M, Acquas E, Di Chiara G. Behavioural sen-

sitization after repeated exposure to Delta 9-tetrahydrocannabinol and cross-sensitization with morphine. *Psychopharmacol.* 2001;158(3):259–266. doi:10.1007/s002130100875.

44. Weisner CM, Campbell CI, Ray GT, et al. Trends in prescribed opioid therapy for non-cancer pain for individuals with prior substance use disorders. *Pain.* 2009;145(3):287–293. doi:10.1016/j.pain.2009.05.006.

45. Beauchamp G, Winstanley EL, Ryan S, Lyons MS. Moving beyond misuse and diversion: the urgent need to consider the role of iatrogenic addiction in the current opioid epidemic. *Am J Public Health.* 2014;104(11):2023–2029. doi:10.2105/AJPH.2014.302147.

46. Porter J, Jick H. Addiction rare in patients treated with narcotics. *N Engl J Med.* 1980;302(2):123.

47. Martell BA, O'Connor PG, Kerns RD, Al E. Systematic review: opioid treatment for chronic back pain: prevalence, efficacy, and association with addiction. *Ann Intern Med.* 2007;146(2):116–127.

48. Wagner FA, Anthony JC. Into the world of illegal drug use: exposure opportunity and other mechanisms linking the use of alcohol, tobacco, marijuana, and cocaine. *Am J Epidemiol.* 2002;155:918–925. doi:10.1093/aje/155.10.918.

49. Kandel DB, Jessor R. The Gateway Hypothesis revisited. In: Kandel DB, ed. *Stages and Pathways of Drug Involvement: Examining the Gateway Hypothesis.* Cambridge: Cambridge University Press; July 2009:365–372.

50. Taub RS. *God of Our Understanding: Jewish Spirituality and Recovery from Addiction.* Jersey City, NJ: KTAV Publishing House; 2011.

51. Crews F, He J, Hodge C. Adolescent cortical development: a critical period of vulnerability for addiction. *Pharmacol Biochem Behav.* 2007;86(2):189–199. doi:10.1016/j.pbb.2006.12.001.

52. Selemon LD. A role for synaptic plasticity in the adolescent development of executive function. *Transl Psychiatry.* 2013;3:e238. doi:10.1038/tp.2013.7.

53. Forman RF, Marlowe DB, McLellan T. The Internet as a source of drugs of abuse. *Curr Psychiatry Rep.* 2006;8(5):377–382. doi:10.1007/s11920-006-0039-6.

54. Walsh C, Phil M. Drugs, the Internet and change. *J Psychoactive Drugs.* 2011;43(March):55–63. doi:10.1080/02791072.2011.56650.

55. The National Center on Addiction and Substance Abuse (CASA). You've Got Drugs! Prescription Drug Pushers on the Internet. 2008. http://www.centeronaddiction.org/addiction-research/reports/youve-got-drugs-prescription-drug-pushers-internet-2008.

56. McCarthy M. Illicit drug use in the US holds steady, but heroin use is on rise. *BMJ.* 2013;347(September):f5544. doi:10.1136/bmj.f5544.

57. Lankenau SE, Teti M, Silva K, Jackson Bloom J, Harocopos A, Treese M. Initiation into prescription opioid misuse amongst young injection drug users. *J Drug Policy.* 2012;23(1):37–44.

58. Cicero TJ, Ellis MS, Surratt HL, Kurtz SP. The changing face of heroin use

in the United States: a retrospective analysis of the past 50 years. *JAMA Psychiatry*. 2014. doi:10.1001/jamapsychiatry.2014.366.

59. Bruner J. Life as narrative. *Soc Res (New York)*. 2004;71:691–711. http://socialresearch.metapress.com/index/e9dffrmjv9aq9xg5.pdf.

60. Hacking I. The looping effects of human kind. In: Sperber D, ed. *Causal Cognition: A Multidisciplinary Debate*. Oxford: Clarendon Press; 1996.

61. Meldrum ML. A capsule history of pain management. *JAMA*. 2003;290(18): 2470–2475. doi:10.1001/jama.290.18.2470.

62. Woolf CJ. Central sensitization: implications for the diagnosis and treatment of pain. *Pain*. 2012;152(3)(suppl):1–31. doi:10.1016/j.pain.2010.09.030 .Central.

63. National Institute on Drug Abuse. Prescription drug abuse. *Res Rep Ser*. 2014. NIH Publication No. 15-4881.

64. Robison LM, Sclar DA, Skaer TL, Galin RS. National trends in the prevalence of attention-deficit/hyperactivity disorder and the prescribing of methylphenidate among school-age children: 1990–1995. *Clin Pediatr (Phila)*. 1999;38(4):209–217. doi:10.1177/000992289903800402.

65. Szasz T. *The Myth of Mental Illness: Foundations of a Theory of Personal Conduct*. New York, NY: Harper Perennial; 1961.

66. Clarke L. Sacred radical of psychiatry. *J Psychiatr Ment Health Nurs*. 2007;14(5):446–453. doi:10.1111/j.1365-2850.2007.01103.x.

67. The diagnostic status of homosexuality in DSM-III: a reformulation of the issues. *Am J Psychiatry*. 1981;138(2):210–215. doi:10.1176/ajp.138.2.210.

68. Luhrmann T. *Of Two Minds: The Growing Disorder in American Psychiatry*. New York, NY: Alfred A Knopf; 2000.

69. Gu Q, Dillon CF, Burt VL. Prescription drug use continues to increase: U.S. prescription drug data for 2007–2008. *NCHS Data Brief*. 2010;No. 42:1–8.

70. Drugfree.org. 2012 Partnership Attitude Tracking Study; 2013. http://www.drugfree.org/wp-content/uploads/2013/04/PATS-2012-FULL-REPORT2.pdf. Accessed December 16, 2013.

71. Garnier-Dykstra LM, Caldeira KM, Vincent KB, O'Grady KE, Arria A. Nonmedical use of prescription stimulants during college: four-year trends in exposure opportunity, use, motives, and sources. *J Am Coll Health*. 2012;60(3):226.

72. Setlik J, Bond GR, Ho M. Adolescent prescription ADHD medication abuse is rising along with prescriptions for these medications. *Pediatrics*. 2009;124(3):875–880. doi:10.1542/peds.2008-0931.

73. Manchikanti L. National drug control policy and prescription drug abuse: facts and fallacies. *Pain Physician*. 2007;10(3):399–424.

74. Smith ME, Farah MJ. Are prescription stimulants "smart pills"? the epidemiology and cognitive neuroscience of prescription stimulant use by normal healthy individuals. *Psychol Bull*. 2011;137(5):717–741. doi:10.1037 /a0023825.

75. Kureishi H. The art of distraction. *New York Times*. February 18, 2012.

76. Lembke A. Time to abandon the self-medication hypothesis in patients with psychiatric disorders. *Am J Drug Alcohol Abuse*. 2012;38(6):524–529. doi:10.3109/00952990.2012.694532.

77. Zimmermann M. [History of pain treatment from 1500 to 1900]. *Schmerz*. 2007;21(4):297–306. doi:10.1007/s00482-007-0573-0.

78. Meldrum ML. *Progress in Pain Research and Management*, V. 25. Seattle, WA: IASP Press; 2003.

79. Agrawal S, Brennan N, Budetti P. The Sunshine Act—effects on physicians. *N Engl J Med*. 2013;368(22):2054–2057. doi:10.1056/NEJMp1303523.

80. Wazana A. Physicians and the pharmaceutical industry: is a gift ever just a gift? *JAMA*. 2000;283(3):373–380. doi.org/10.1001/jama.283.3.373. http://dx.doi.org/10.1001/jama.283.3.373.

81. Meier B. *Pain Killer: A Wonder Drug's Trail of Addiction and Death*. New York, NY: St. Martin's Press; 2003.

82. Hegmann KT, Weiss MS, Bowden K, et al. ACOEM practice guidelines: opioids for treatment of acute, subacute, chronic, and postoperative pain. *JOEM*. 2014;56(12):143–159. doi:10.1097/JOM.0000000000000352.

83. Agency for Healthcare Research and Quality. The effectiveness and risks of long-term opioid treatment of chronic pain. *Evid Rep Technol Assess*. 2014;No. 218. http://www.ncbi.nlm.nih.gov/books/NBK258809/.

84. Lee M, Silverman SM, Hansen H, Patel VB, Manchikanti L. A comprehensive review of opioid-induced hyperalgesia. *Pain Physician*. 2011;14(2):145–161. http://www.ncbi.nlm.nih.gov/pubmed/21412369.

85. Chu LF, Clark DJ, Angst MS. Opioid tolerance and hyperalgesia in chronic pain patients after one month of oral morphine therapy: a preliminary prospective study. *J Pain*. 2006;7(1):43–48. doi:10.1016/j.jpain.2005.08.001.

86. Portenoy RK, Foley KM. Chronic use of opioid analgesics in non-malignant pain: report of 38 cases. *Pain*. 1986;25(2):171–186.

87. Sullivan MD, Howe CQ. Opioid therapy for chronic pain in the United States: promises and perils. *Pain*. 2013;154(suppl):S94–S100. doi:10.1016/j.pain.2013.09.009.

88. Weissman DE, Haddox JD. Opioid pseudoaddiction—an iatrogenic syndrome. *Pain*. 1989;36:363–366.

89. Live interview with Dr. Russell Portenoy. *Physicians Responsible Opioid Prescribing*. https://www.youtube.com/watch?v=DgyuBWN9D4w. Accessed September 2, 2015.

90. Ornstein C, Weber T. American Pain Foundation shuts down as senators launch an investigation of prescription narcotics. *ProPublica*, May 8, 2012. https://www.propublica.org/article/senate-panel-investigates-drug-company-ties-to-pain-groups. Accessed March 20, 2016.

91. The use of opioids for the treatment of chronic pain: a consensus statement from the American Academy of Pain Medicine and the American Pain Society. *Clin J Pain*. 1997;13(1).

92. Pizzo P. Relieving pain in America: a blueprint for transforming preven-

tion, care, education, and research. *Inst Med.* June 2011:382. doi:10.3109/1 5360288.2012.678473.

93. Manchikanti L, Singh A. Therapeutic opioids: a ten-year perspective on the complexities and complications of the escalating use, abuse, and nonmedical use of opioids. *Pain Physician.* 2008;11:S63–S88.

94. International Association for the Study of Pain. Declaration that access to pain management is a fundamental human right. *Declaration of Montreal.* http://www.iasp-pain.org/DeclarationofMontreal. Accessed September 2, 2015.

95. The Joint Commission. http://www.jointcommission.org/. Accessed September 2, 2015.

96. Vila HJ, Smith RA, Augustyniak MJ. The efficacy and safety of pain management before and after implementation of hospital-wide pain management standards: is patient safety compromised by treatment based solely on numerical pain ratings? *Anesth Analg.* 2005;101:474–480.

97. Frasco PE, Sprung J, Trentman TL. The impact of The Joint Commission for accreditation of healthcare organizations pain initiative on perioperative opiate consumption and recovery room length of stay. *Anesth Analg.* 2005;100:162–168.

98. GAO. Prescription OxyContin abuse and diversion and efforts to address the problem. *J Pain Palliat Care Pharmacother.* 2003;18(3):109–113. doi:10 .1300/J354v18n03_12.

99. Catan T, Perez E. A pain drug champion has second thoughts. *Wall Street Journal.* December 17, 2012.

100. The Joint Commission. Sentinel Event Alert Issue 49: Safe use of opioids in hospitals. http://www.jointcommission.org/sea_issue_49/.

101. Fauber J. FDA and pharma: emails raise pay-for-play concerns. *Sentinal/ MedPage Today.* http://www.medpagetoday.com/PainManagement/Pain Management/42103.

102. Juurlink DN, Dhalla IA, Nelson LS. Improving opioid prescribing: the New York City recommendations. *JAMA.* 2013;309(9):879–880.

103. Armstrong D. Suit over OxyContin—could be painful. *Bloomberg Business.* http://www.bloomberg.com/news/articles/2014-10-20/purdue-says-ken tucky-suit-over-oxycontin-could-be-painful.

104. McDonald DC, Carlson KE. Estimating the prevalence of opioid diversion by "doctor shoppers" in the United States. *PLoS One.* 2013;8(7):e69241. doi: 10.1371/journal.pone.0069241.

105. Dole VP, Nyswander ME. Heroin addiction—a metabolic disease. *Arch Intern Med.* 1967;120(1):19–24. http://dx.doi.org/10.1001/archinte.1967.003 00010021004.

106. Strang J, Babor T, Caulkins J, Fischer B, Foxcroft D, Humphreys K. Drug policy and the public good: evidence for effective interventions. *Lancet.* 2012;379(9810):71–83. doi:10.1016/S0140-6736(11)61674-7.

107. Gjersing L, Bretteville-Jensen AL. Is opioid substitution treatment ben-

eficial if injecting behaviour continues? *Drug Alcohol Depend.* 2013;133: 121–126.

108. Lynch FL, McCarty D, Mertens J, et al. Costs of care for persons with opioid dependence in commercial integrated health systems. *Addict Sci Clin Pract.* 2014;9(1):16. doi:10.1186/1940-0640-9-16.

109. Lofwall MR, Martin J, Tierney M, Fatséas M, Auriacombe M, Lintzeris N. Buprenorphine diversion and misuse in outpatient practice. *J Addict Med.* 2014;8(5):327–332. doi:10.1097/ADM.0000000000000029.

110. Axelrod R. *The Evolution of Cooperation.* New York, NY: Basic Books Inc; 1984.

111. Axelrod R. Effective choice in the prisoner's dilemma. *J Conflict Resolut.* 1980;24(1):3–25.

112. Parsons T. The sick role and the role of the physician reconsidered. *Millbank Mem Fund Q Health Soc.* 1975;53(3):257–278.

113. Autor DH, Duggan MG. The growth in the Social Security disability rolls: a fiscal crisis unfolding. *J Econ Perspect.* 2006;20(3):71–96.

114. Laffaye C, Rosen CS, Schnurr PP, Friedman MJ. Does compensation status influence treatment participation and course of recovery from posttraumatic stress disorder? *Mil Med.* 2007;172(10):1039–1045.

115. Angrist JD, Chen SH, Frandsen BR. Did Vietnam veterans get sicker in the 1990s? The complicated effects of military service on self-reported health. *J Public Econ.* 2010;94:824–837.

116. Rosenheck R, Fontana AF. Recent trends in VA treatment of post-traumatic stress disorder and other mental disorders. *Health Aff.* 2007;26:1720–1727.

117. Wen P. A legacy of unintended side effects. *Boston Globe.* December 12, 2010.

118. Fassin D, Rechtman R. *The Empire of Trauma: An Inquiry into the Condition of Victimhood.* Princeton, NJ: Princeton University Press; 2009.

119. Mack K, Zhang K, Paulozzi L, Jones C. Prescription practices involving opioid analgesics among Americans with Medicaid, 2010. *J Health Care Poor Underserved.* 2015;26(1):182–198. doi:10.1353/hpu.2015.0009.

120. Frueh BC, Grubaugh AL, Elhai JD, Buckley TD. US Department of Veterans Affairs Disability policies for posttraumatic stress disorder: administrative trends and implications for treatment, rehabilitation, and research. *Am J Public Health* 2007;97(12):2143–2145.

121. Seal KH, Shi Y, Cohen G, et al. Association of mental health disorders with prescription opioids and high-risk opioid use in US veterans of Iraq and Afghanistan. *JAMA.* 2012;307(9):940–947.

122. Wilkinson R, Marmot M. *Social Determinants of Health: The Solid Facts.* 2nd ed. Copenhagen: World Health Organization; 2003.

123. Davis JE. Victim narratives and victim selves: false memory sydrome and the power of accounts. *Soc Probl.* 2005;52(4):529–548.

124. Hacking I. Making up people. *London Rev Books.* 2006;28(16).

125. Children and Adults with Attention Deficit Disorder (CHADD). www.chadd.org. Accessed August 1, 2015.

126. Autor D, Duggan M. Supporting work: a proposal for modernizing the US disability insurance system. *Cent Am Prog Hamilt Proj.* December 2010. http://scholar.google.com/scholar?hl=en&btnG=Search&q=intitle:Supporting+Work+:+A+Proposal+for+Modernizing+the+U.S.+Disability+Insurance+System#0\nhttp://www.americanprogress.org/wp-content/uploads/issues/2010/12/pdf/autordugganpaper.pdf.

127. Kohut H. *The Kohut Seminars: On Self Psychology and Psychotherapy with Adolescents and Young Adults* (Elson M, ed.). New York, NY: W W Norton; 1987.

128. Buber M. *I and Thou.* New York, NY: Charles Scribner's Sons; 1937.

129. Vaillant GE, Bond M, Vaillant CO. An empirically validated hierarchy of defense mechanisms. *Arch Gen Psychiatry.* 1986;43(8):786–794.

130. Perrone J, Nelson LS. Medication reconciliation for controlled substances—an "ideal" prescription-drug monitoring program. *N Engl J Med.* 2012;366(25):2341–2343. doi:10.1056/NEJMp1204493.

131. Center of Excellence Brandeis University Briefing on PDMP Effectiveness; 2013. www.pdmpexcellence.org.

132. Compton WM, Jones CM, Baldwin GT. Relationship between nonmedical prescription-opioid use and heroin use. *N Engl J Med.* 2016;374:154–163.

133. Silvestrini E. Florida heals from pill mill epidemic. *Tampa Tribune.* August 30, 2014.

134. Imai M. *Kaizen: The Key to Japan's Competitive Success.* New York, NY: McGraw-Hill Education; 1986.

135. Deaton JP. How automotive production lines work. *HowStuffWorks.com.* http://auto.howstuffworks.com/under-the-hood/auto-manufacturing/automotive-production-line.htm. Accessed June 6, 2015.

136. Kocher R, Sahni N. Hospitals' race to employ physicians—the logic behind a money-losing proposition. *N Engl J Med.* 2011:1790–1793.

137. Sinsky CA, Dugdale DC. Medicare payment for cognitive vs procedural care: minding the gap. *JAMA Intern Med.* 2013.

138. Williams B. Patient satisfaction: a valid concept? *Soc Sci Med.* 1994;38(4):509–516.

139. Press Ganey. http://www.pressganey.com/. Accessed September 9, 2015.

140. Fenton JJ, Jerant F, Bertakis KD, Franks P. The cost of satisfaction: a national study of patient satisfaction, health care utilization, expenditures, and mortality. *Arch Intern Med.* 2012;172(5):405–411. doi:10.1001/archinternmed.2011.1662.

141. Nelson EC, Larson C. Patients' good and bad surprises: how do they relate to overall patient satisfaction? *Qual Rev Bull.* 1993;3(89).

142. King R. Obamacare program may be linked to ER opioid prescriptions. *Washington Examiner.* May 7, 2015.

143. Frankt AB, Bagley N. Protection or harm? supressing substance use data. *N Engl J Med.* 2015 May 14;372(20):1879–1881.

144. Chen JH, Humphreys K, Shah NH, Lembke A. Distribution of opioids by different types of medicare prescribers. *JAMA Intern Med.* December 2015:1–3. http://dx.doi.org/10.1001/jamainternmed.2015.6662.

145. Rush B. *An Inquiry Into the Effects of Ardent Spirits Upon the Human Body and Mind: With an Account of the Means of Preventing, and of the Remedies for Curing Them.* Exeter, NH: Josiah Richardson Bookseller; 1819.

146. White WL. *Slaying the Dragon: The History of Addiction Treatment and Recovery in America.* Bloomington, IL: Chestnut Health Systems; 1998.

147. The National Center on Addiction and Substance Abuse. Addiction medicine: closing the gap between science and practice; 2012. http://www.cen teronaddiction.org/addiction-research/reports/addiction-medicine.

148. McLellan AT, Lewis DC, O'Brien CP, Kleber HD. Drug dependence, a chronic medical illness: implications for treatment, insurance, and outcomes evaluation. *JAMA.* 2000;284:1689–1695. doi:10.1001/jama.284.13.1689.

149. Umberg EN, Shader RI, Hsu LKG, Greenblatt DJ. From disordered eating to addiction: the "food drug" in bulimia nervosa. *J Clin Psychopharmacol.* 2012;32:376–389. doi:10.1097/00132586-200108000-00061.

150. Hernandez L, Hoebel BG. Food reward and cocaine increase extracellular dopamine in the nucleus accumbens as measured by microdialysis. *Life Sci.* 1988;42:1705–1712. doi:10.1016/0024-3205(88)90036-7.

151. Avena NM, Bocarsly ME. Dysregulation of brain reward systems in eating disorders: neurochemical information from animal models of binge eating, bulimia nervosa, and anorexia nervosa. *Neuropharmacol.* 2012;63:87–96. doi:10.1016/j.neuropharm.2011.11.010.

152. Duhigg C. *The Power of Habit: Why We Do What We Do in Life and Business.* New York, NY: Random House; 2012.

153. Ahmed SH. Imbalance between drug and non-drug reward availability: a major risk factor for addiction. *Eur J Pharmacol.* 2005;526(1–3):9–20. doi:10.1016/j.ejphar.2005.09.036.

154. Campbell UC, Carroll ME. Acquisition of drug self-administration: environmental and pharmacological interventions. *Exp Clin Psychopharmacol.* 2000;8:312–325. doi:10.1037/1064-1297.8.3.312.

155. Fischer B, Rehm J, Patra J, Firestone CM. Changes in illicit opioid use profiles across Canada. *CMAJ.* 2006;175:1–3.

156. Davis W, Johnson B. Prescription opioid use, misuse, and diversion among street drug users in New York City. *Drug Alcohol Depend.* 2008;92:267–276.

157. Drury B, Gelzer R, Trites P, Paul GT. Electronic health records systems: testing the limits of digital records' reliability and trust. *Ave Maria Law Rev.* 2014:257–276.

158. Humphreys K. An overdose antidote goes mainstream. *Health Aff.* 2015; 34(10):1624–1627. doi:10.1377/hlthaff.2015.0934.

159. Rudd RA, Aleshire N, Zibbell JE, Gladden RM. Increases in drug and opioid overdose deaths—United States, 2000–2014. *MMWR Morb Mortal Wkly Rep.* 2016;64:1378–1382. http://www.cdc.gov/mmwr/preview/mmwrhtml /mm6450a3.htm.

160. Wood E, Samet JH, Volkow ND. Physician education in addiction medicine. *JAMA.* 2013;310(16):1673–1674. doi:10.1001/jama.2013.280377.

Index

AA (Alcoholics Anonymous), 13, 18–19, 99–100
academic physicians, role of, in epidemic, 57–62
ADD (attention deficit disorder), 45–46, 49
Adderall, 45–46, 49–52
addiction: to benzodiazepines, 145–46; bulimia and, 137; consequences of, 14, 134–35, 142–45; diagnostic criteria for, 14; drug-seeking patients and, 79–80; eating disorders and, 137; gateway hypothesis of, 22–23; to heroin, 30–33; Portenoy on rates of, 61; recovery from, 18–19, 134; reward circuitry of brain and, 15, 22, 137; risk for, 16–18, 24, 95–97, 138; sharing of information about, 126–27; terminology, xi, 14n. *See also* addiction treatment; models of addiction; opioid addiction; substance use disorder; withdrawal
addiction treatment: chronic care model of, 153–54; Drug Addiction Treatment Act, 84; insurance companies and, 131–32, 134; training in, 152–53
adolescents. *See* teens and prescription drugs
advertising, direct-to-consumer, 58n
Affordable Care Act, 134
Alcoholics Anonymous (AA), 13, 18–19, 99–100
alcohol withdrawal, 127–28
alternative rewards, as reducing substance use, 138
American Academy of Pain Medicine, 63

American Pain Foundation, 62–63
American Pain Society, 63
antidepressants, for adults, 48
anxiety, and defense mechanisms, 106–8
"Art of Distraction, The" (Kureishi), 50
assessment of pain, 66
attention deficit disorder (ADD), 45–46, 49
autism spectrum disorders, 98
autobiographical narratives, 39–40
Autor, David, 91, 92, 101
Axelrod, Robert, 87

BAART (Bay Area Addiction Research and Treatment), 33
backward logic in mental health care field, 46
benzodiazepines: addiction to, 145–46; combination of opioids and, 4; as schedule IV drugs, 6
Bergman v. Eden Medical Center, 64
best practices, 65–66
Big Medicine, role of, in epidemic: academic physicians, 57–62; FDA, 67–71; Federation of State Medical Boards, 64–65; professional medical societies, 62–64
Big Pharma: academic physicians and, 58–62; class actions suits against, 71; FDA and, 68; JCAHO and, 67; opioid epidemic and, 57; "pain management educational program" for hospitals and, 66–67; perks given to doctors by, 57–58; professional medical societies and, 62–63

brain pathology, individual difference as, 43–49
Bruner, Jerome, 40
Buber, Martin, 105
bulimia nervosa, 136–37
bullies, 78

case studies: Diana, 135–48; Justin, 23–25, 26–28, 29, 30, 32–36; Karen, 44–46, 49–53; Macy, 109–13; opioid addiction, 3–4; overview of, 7; Sally, 89–90, 97, 100. *See also* Jim case study
Centers for Disease Control and Prevention (CDC), 3
Centers for Medicare and Medicaid Services (CMS), 65, 124–25, 127
central sensitization, 43
CHADD, 98
"chasing the dragon," 32
childhood trauma: addiction risk and, 17; psychopathology and, 41
chronic care model of addiction treatment, 153–54
chronic pain syndromes: disability claims for, 92; FDA and clinical trials of drugs for, 68–70; as growing problem, 42–43; new models for care of, 154–55; opioids for management of, 59–61
Clarke, L., 47
clinical trials of drugs, 68–70
CMS (Centers for Medicare and Medicaid Services), 65, 124–25, 127
cocaine, 140
communication between doctors, 126–28
compassionate doctors, 104–8
compulsion and addiction, 14
consequences of addiction, 14, 134–35, 142–45
contingency management, 88
control and addiction, 14
controlled prescription drugs: online pharmacies and, 28, 29; types of, 5–7
Controlled Substance Act (CSA), 5, 28
country mice and city mice, 77–78
cross-sensitization or cross-addiction, 21–22

culture: addiction and, 15–16; autobiographical narratives and, 40
cyberpharmacies, 27–30

Dannemiller Foundation, 59
DARE (Drug Abuse Resistance Education), 25n
Davis, Joseph, 97
DAWN (Drug Abuse Warning Network), 6
"deep web," 30
defense mechanisms, 106–8
denial: of addiction, 85–86; as defense mechanism, 107–8
destigmatization of opioid therapy, campaign for, 58–64
Diagnostic and Statistical Manual of Mental Disorders (DSM), 14, 79
difference, as psychopathology, 43–49
direct-to-consumer advertising, 58n
disease model of addiction, 133–35
doctors: as baristas, 128–29; as compassionate, 104–8; as corrupt, 115–18; perks given to, by Big Pharma, 57–58; prescribing practices of, 56–57, 58n, 64; prisoners' dilemma for, 86–88. *See also* overprescribing; psychiatrists
doctor shopping, 74, 77
Dole, Vincent, 82–83
dopamine, 80–81, 137
dose of opioids, 60
Drug Abuse Resistance Education (DARE), 25n
Drug Abuse Warning Network (DAWN), 6
Drug Addiction Treatment Act of 2000, 84
Drug Enforcement Agency, 103
drugs. *See* prescription drugs; *and specific drugs*
drug-seeking behavior: addiction and, 79–80; case study, 73–75; compassionate doctors and, 106–8; denial and, 85–86; malingering and, 79; methadone maintenance and, 83; prisoners' dilemma for doctors and, 86–88; as pseudoaddiction, 61; strategies, 75–79
DSM (Diagnostic and Statistical Manual of Mental Disorders), 14, 79

Duggan, Mark, 91, 92, 101
Duhigg, Charles, 138
Dynamic Duos, 77
"dysphoria-driven" relapse, 81

eating disorders and addiction, 137
electronic medical records, 145
emotion dysregulation, 16–17
endorphins, 3n, 137
enriched enrollment study protocol, 68–70
epidemics: opioid, in U.S., 57n; prescription drug, 4–5, 25–27, 128. *See also* Big Medicine, role of, in epidemic
exhibitionists, 76

Fassin, D., 97
Fauber, John, 68
FDA (Food and Drug Administration), 5–7, 67–71
Federation of State Medical Boards, role of, in epidemic, 64–65
fellowships in addiction medicine, 153
financial incentives and patient satisfaction, 124–25
Florida, pill mills in, 118
Foley, Kathleen, 60–61
Food and Drug Administration (FDA), 5–7, 67–71
42CFR Part 2, 126–28
Forman, R. F., 28
Freud, Sigmund, 41, 105, 106
Frueh, B. C., 100–101

Ganey, Rod, 123
gateway hypothesis of addiction, 22–23
Gawehn, Barbara, 154–55
genetic risk for addiction, 16–17
Good Samaritan laws, 150

Hacking, Ian, 41, 98
Haddox, David, 65
Harrison Narcotic Act of 1914, 31
heroin: addiction to, 30–33; complications of use of, 142–45; epidemics of, 57n; as illicit source of opioids, 109; recovery from, 33–35; types of, 140–41

"heroin chic" in Manhattan, 139
hijacked brain model of addiction, 79–82
Hoffmann, Felix, 31
homosexuality, as mental illness, 47
hospice care, 57
Hospital Consumer Assessment of Healthcare Providers and Systems survey, 124–25
hospitals: electronic health records and, 145; eligibility service providers and, 94; 42CFR Part 2 and, 127–28; incentive-based compensation for staff of, 122; opioid addiction and, 2–3, 21, 39–40, 55–56, 110–11, 143; physician practices owned by, 119–20; quality measures of, 124–25
hydrocodone (Vicodin), 5–6, 24–25, 70–71

Iacono, W. G., 16–17
illness identity, 97–100
illness narratives: centralized pain syndromes, 41–43; difference is psychopathology, 43–49; drug-seeking behavior and, 85–86; overview of, 39–40; pain as dangerous, 40–41; shaping, 155
impersonators, 77
impulsivity, 16–17
incentive-based compensation, 122
industrialization of medical care, 118–26
Institute of Medicine committee, "Relieving Pain in America" report of, 63
insurance companies and addiction treatment, 131–32, 134
integrated health care systems, 119–20, 126
International Association for the Study of Pain, 63–64
Internet copycats, 78

James v. Hillhaven, 64
Jewish people and addiction, 23
Jim case study: AA experience, 12–14; career and leisure, 10–12, 13; drug-seeking behavior, 73–75, 89, 103–4, 115–17; early life, 9–10; follow-up after treatment, 149–50; opioid addiction, 21, 39–40, 55–56; opioid treatment, 131–32

Parsons, Talcott, 91
Passik, Steven, 109
passive aggression, 106–7
patient advocacy groups, 98
patient satisfaction surveys, 123–26
PDMP (Prescription Drug Monitoring Program), 103, 107–8, 150
peer influence, 17
Penandpaper.com, 35
Peters, Karen, 154–55
pharmaceutical industry. *See* Big Pharma
physician assistants, 153
physicians. *See* doctors; psychiatrists
physiologic dependence and withdrawal, 14–15
pill mills, 115–18
Pipemania.com, 29
placebo in clinical trials of drugs, 68–69
pleasure-pain balance, 80–82
Portenoy, Russell, 59–62, 63
post-traumatic stress disorder (PTSD), 41, 92, 93, 95, 96
poverty, medicalization of, 93–95
Power of Habit, The (Duhigg), 138
prescription drug epidemic, 4–5, 25–27, 128. *See also* Big Medicine, role of, in epidemic
Prescription Drug Monitoring Program (PDMP), 103, 107–8, 150
prescription drugs: availability of, 17–18; controlled or scheduled, 5–7, 28, 29; for individual differences, 45–47; misuse of, 2–3, 18, 25–26, 48–49; spending for, 48; teens and, 23–25, 26–27, 36–37, 48–49. *See also* drug-seeking behavior; overdoses; prescription drug epidemic; research; *and specific drugs*
Press, Irwin, 123
prisoners' dilemma for doctors, 86–88
professional medical societies, role of, in epidemic, 62–64
professional patients: case study, 89–90, 146–47; description of, 90–91; illness identity and victim narrative of, 97–100; medicalization of poverty and, 93–95; risk for addiction in, 95–97; SSDI and, 90–93, 100–101

projection, 107
pseudoaddiction, 61
psychiatrists, 47–48, 121
psychological trauma, 41
PTSD (post-traumatic stress disorder), 41, 92, 93, 95, 96
Purdue Pharma, 57, 63, 64–65, 67, 71
Purple Drank, 29–30

quality measures, 124

Rapoport, Anatol, 87
Rechtman, R., 97
recovery from addiction, 18–19, 134
recovery movement, 99–100
refusal to treat addicted patients, 108–13
reinstatement, 21–22
relapse, 21–22, 81
Relative Value Units, 121
"Relieving Pain in America" (Institute of Medicine committee report), 63
research: of academic physicians, 58–62; clinical trials of drugs, 68–70
"research chemicals," 29
reward circuitry of brain, 15, 22, 137
rewards, alternative, as reducing substance use, 138
risk for addiction, 16–18, 24, 95–97, 138
role-playing tabletop games, 35–36
Rush, Benjamin, 133

schedule I drugs, 5, 31
schedule II drugs, 5–6, 45, 70
schedule III drugs, 6
schedule IV drugs, 6
schedule V drugs, 6
school-based prevention programs, 25n
sedatives: overprescribing of, 150n; prescriptions of, 4; as schedule IV drugs, 6
Senators, 76
side effects of opioids and dose, 60
Silk Road website, 30
social networks, AA as changing, 19
social roles, 91, 98
Social Security Disability Income (SSDI): increases in claims for, 91–93; professional patients and, 90–91, 100–101